# Arts Therapies Research and I
# with Persons on the Autism Spectrum

This volume presents cutting-edge research and practice on Creative Arts Therapies or Arts Therapies for individuals on the autism spectrum of all ages, outlining the development of effective and accessible approaches to support the diverse needs of this client group.

Consisting of 14 research-based chapters with contributions from over 30 authors from across the world, the book brings together research from art, music, drama, dance, movement and other forms of art therapies. The book demonstrates how arts therapies have evolved over the years to address the health and social care needs of people on the autism spectrum and their caregivers. Chapters explore the implications of arts therapies across a spectrum of needs in various settings and offer a comprehensive picture including a variety of research outcomes and therapeutic processes, and critiques both of existing practice and research methodologies.

The book will be key reading for researchers, scholars and clinicians from dance movement therapy, music therapy, art therapy, dramatherapy and expressive arts therapies. It will also be of interest to post-graduate students and mental health professionals working with children, adults and families of individuals on the autism spectrum.

**Supritha Aithal** is Researcher and Senior Lecturer in Creative Approaches to Psychotherapy, Edge Hill University, UK.

**Vicky Karkou** is Creative Psychotherapist and Professor in Arts and Wellbeing, Edge Hill University, UK.

# International Research in the Arts Therapies

Series Editors: Diane Waller and Sarah Scoble
*A collaboration between* **ECArTE** *(European Consortium for Arts Therapies Education) and* **ICRA** *(International Centre for Research in Arts Therapies, Imperial College, London)*

This series consists of high-level monographs identifying areas of importance across all arts therapy modalities (art therapy, dance movement therapy, dramatherapy and music therapy) and highlighting international developments and concerns. It presents recent research from countries across the world and contributes to the evidence-base of the arts therapies. Papers which discuss and analyse current innovations and approaches in the arts therapies and arts therapy education are also included.

This series is accessible to practitioners of the arts therapies and to colleagues in a broad range of related professions, including those in countries where arts therapies are still emerging. The monographs should also provide a valuable source of reference to government departments and health services.

**Titles in the Series**

For more information about the series, please visit: https://www.routledge.com/International-Research-in-the-Arts-Therapies/book-series/IRAT

# Arts Therapies Research and Practice with Persons on the Autism Spectrum

Colourful Hatchlings

**Edited by Supritha Aithal and Vicky Karkou**

Routledge
Taylor & Francis Group

LONDON AND NEW YORK

Designed cover image: Colourful hatchlings as envisioned by
Apoorva Chakraverthy N (14 years), Sarayu Kala Kuteera, Bengaluru

First published 2024
by Routledge
4 Park Square, Milton Park, Abingdon, Oxon OX14 4RN

and by Routledge
605 Third Avenue, New York, NY 10158

*Routledge is an imprint of the Taylor & Francis Group, an informa business*

*British Library Cataloguing-in-Publication Data*
A catalogue record for this book is available from the British Library

*Library of Congress Cataloguing-in-Publication Data*
Names: Aithal, Supritha, editor. | Karkou, Vassiliki, editor.
Title: Arts therapies research and practice with persons on the autism
spectrum : colourful hatchlings / edited by Supritha Aithal and Vicky Karkou.
Description: New York : Routledge, 2024. | Series: International research in
the arts therapies | Includes bibliographical references and index. |
Identifiers: LCCN 2023014800 (print) | LCCN 2023014801 (ebook) | ISBN
9781032063089 (hardback) | ISBN 9781032063102 (paperback) | ISBN
9781003201656 (ebook)
Subjects: LCSH: Autism spectrum disorders--Treatment. |
Arts--Therapeutic use.
Classification: LCC RC553.A88 A4879 2024 (print) | LCC RC553.A88
(ebook) | DDC 616.85/88206--dc23/eng/20230705
LC record available at https://lccn.loc.gov/2023014800
LC ebook record available at https://lccn.loc.gov/2023014801

ISBN: 978-1-032-06308-9 (hbk)
ISBN: 978-1-032-06310-2 (pbk)
ISBN: 978-1-003-20165-6 (ebk)

DOI: 10.4324/9781003201656

Typeset in Sabon
by MPS Limited, Dehradun

This book is dedicated to the memory of Roger Arguile (1952–2022) who from the 1980s pioneered art therapy with autistic young people in the UK. We were delighted that Roger was able to contribute to this book through an interview that focussed on his life-long practice and research.

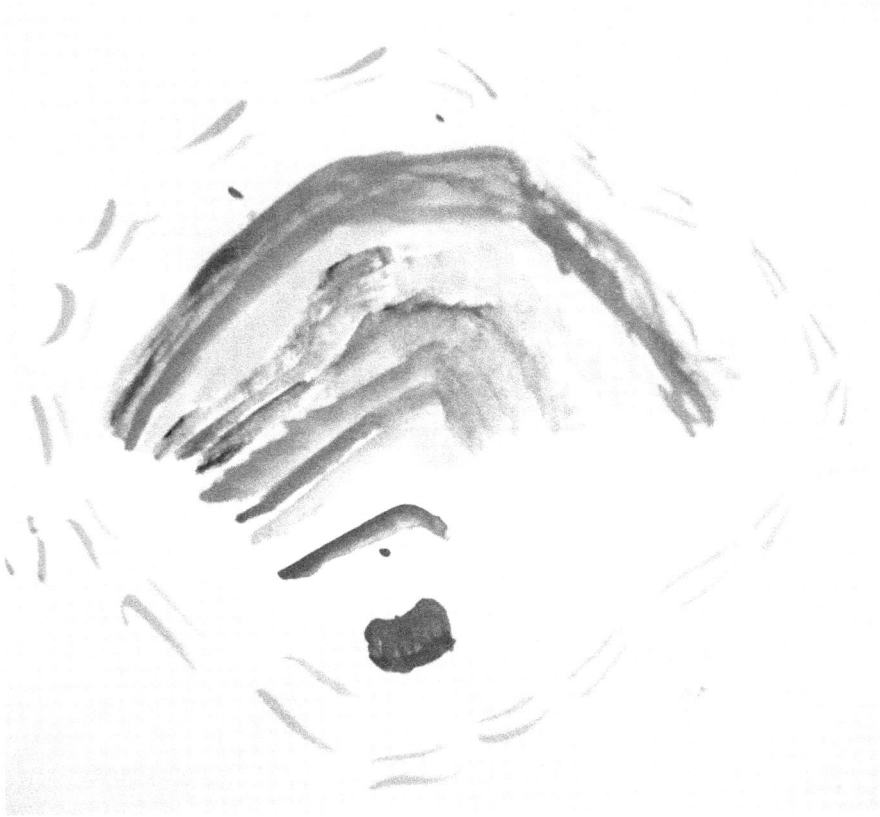

*Figure A* Artwork by Ina Bhamati Kothari (six years), Mysuru

# Contents

# Figures

# Tables

# About the Editors and Contributors

**Supritha Aithal,** PhD, Fellow of the Higher Education Academy, is currently working as a senior lecturer at the Faculty of Health, Social Care and Medicine, Edge Hill University, UK. Passion towards dance and working experience as a speech and language therapist made her step into the field of dance movement psychotherapy (DMP). Supritha joined Edge Hill University as a graduate teaching assistant with a full scholarship to carry out doctoral research and was awarded a PhD in 2020 for her research on the contribution of DMP towards the wellbeing of children with an autism spectrum disorder and their caregivers. Supritha has disseminated her research in various international peer-reviewed journals and international conferences across the globe. She is a recipient of the American Dance Therapy Association's Research Award 2022.

**Sònia Barrachina,** BA, MA, is a freelance HCPC registered dramatherapist with a BA in primary education and MA in educational pedagogy (University of Girona). Sonia studied for her MA in drama and movement therapy at the Royal Central School of Speech and Drama in March 2005 and later a Diploma in Creative Approaches to Supervision at the London Centre for Psychodrama in August 2016. Sonia's work focuses on children with behavioural and emotional difficulties in mainstream primary schools and with elderly adults with moderate to profound Learning Disabilities and Complex Needs. Sonia's specialist area of interest and expertise is in the use of Storytelling with clients with profound and multiple learning disabilities (PMLD).

**Laura Blauth,** PhD, has worked as a music therapist with children, adults and families in various settings, including schools, child development centres, psychiatric units and community settings. In 2019, she obtained her PhD at Anglia Ruskin University, Cambridge, investigating the effects of music therapy and parent counselling on resilience in young children with autism and their families. She is passionate about family-centred and strength-based music therapy approaches, and about working collaboratively with professionals from other disciplines. Laura is currently a research fellow at the University of Applied Sciences in Würzburg (Germany) within HOMESIDE, an international RCT on music therapy, dementia and family caregivers. She presents her research and clinical work at international conferences and in books and journals.

**Loukia Bololia,** PhD, has extensive professional experience working as a psychopedagogist and is an HCPC registered dramatherapist primarily with children and young people with developmental conditions and complex needs in educational, community and clinical settings. She holds an interdisciplinary BSc in philosophy and social studies (namely, pedagogy and psychology) and an MSc in child, adolescent and family mental health. Her passion for arts-based psychotherapy guided her to undertake a postgraduate training in Dramatherapy. Her clinical practice has an integrative orientation, concentrating on child holistic development, mental health promotion and wellbeing, social sensitisation and pedagogical culture of creativity. Loukia completed her PhD in clinical and health psychology at the University of Edinburgh, and her research focused on Dramatherapy and adolescents on the autism spectrum. She is currently a lecturer and supervisor within the frame of developmental and psychological science in Higher Education in the UK.

**Emeline Brulé,** PhD, is a lecturer at the University of Sussex (UK). Initially trained as a designer, they received a PhD in communication studies from Télécom ParisTech for their ethnographic work on the experiences of schooling of visually impaired children and their design work on learning technologies for this group. Emeline Brulé currently studies design and organisational processes behind digital products, focusing on the areas of education technologies, assistive technologies and technologies for the home.

**Lynn Cedar** co-founded Roundabout, the largest Dramatherapy charity in the UK in the mid-1980s where she is an experienced fundraiser, manager and practitioner. Lynn is a specialist in working with elderly adults and with children and young people with learning disabilities. She is also an experienced clinical supervisor. Her publications include the journal article "Roundabout and the Big Lottery: A Four Year Dramatherapy Project for Older Adults" (2016) and the book *Child Agency and Voice in Therapy: New Ways of Working in the Arts Therapies* (2020).

**Christina Devereaux,** PhD, LCAT, LMHC, BC-DMT, is associate clinical professor and program director for the Dance/Movement Therapy and Counseling programme at Drexel University in the College of Nursing and Health Professions. She served as co-editor for the *American Journal* *of Dance Therapy* 2011–2017 and received the ADTA President's award in 2010 and 2017 for her contributions to the profession.

**Lidia Atencia-Doña**, PhD, BA, currently works as assistant professor at the Dance Conservatory of Malaga (Spain). With an active professional life as a dancer, Lidia has collaborated with some of the most renowned dance companies in Spain, being awarded international prizes. Lidia's publications comprise of those in journals such as *The Arts in Psychotherapy and Danzaratte*, as well as in the proceedings of the II International Conference on Dance, Research and Education (University of Malaga). She has been a speaker on dance education and dance therapy for different educational institutions, and regularly contributes as a volunteer to the care institution Centro Pinares de Autism, leading free-to-all sessions of dance and music-therapy since 2008.

**Huma Durrani**, RCAT, RP(Qualifying), DAT, MAAT, is a Pakistani Singaporean who is self-employed as an art therapist. She has professional and personal experience of almost two decades working with children and adolescents with differences, first as an educational therapist and then as an art therapist. Huma has conducted doctoral research on ASD and comorbid SID that she has published in academic journals and presented internationally. She designed a framework for doing art therapy with children with autism, documented in her book *Sensory-Based Relational Art Therapy Approach (S-BRATA): Supporting Psycho-Emotional Needs in Children with Autism*. Huma has also published a memoir called *Wrapped in Blue* in which she documented her journey about raising her son with autism.

**Nicky Dyer** has an MA in Dramatherapy (Roehampton University) a diploma in the arts and initially trained as a dance and drama teacher and worked for over 27 years in both mainstream and special schools. She is an HCPC registered freelance dramatherapist and has worked both in mainstream primary and secondary schools with young people of all ages who have a wide range of issues. She has been specifically involved with young people on the autistic spectrum, working with a local autistic charity, and led the autistic support in a local primary school for four years. She also runs a private practice. In 2017, she had an article published in the *Dramatherapy Journal* on her work with children on the autistic spectrum.

**Xavier Fontenille**, MA Dramatherapy, before training as a dramatherapist, Xavier trained as an actor at Drama Studio London 2001. He began working for Roundabout that same year. Currently, Xavier is working with children who are on the autistic spectrum, as well as those who have emotional/behavioural issues, and those who have ADHD. Autism has become a particular interest for him. He has pursued this through further training with the Caldwell Foundation, learning the techniques of Intensive Interaction. Xavier has also completed Level 2 training in Sherborne Developmental Movement.

**Andrea Gleason,** MA, is a registered psychologist in the province of Alberta, Canada and a graduate of the McGill Counselling Program in Montreal, Canada. She has worked with children and adults in various capacities, including classroom and family consultation, assessment, counselling and Dance Movement Therapy. She is in the process of becoming a registered dance/movement therapist with the American Dance Therapy Association through the Alternate Route training.

**Judith Good,** PhD, is professor of human-computer interaction in the Informatics Institute at the University of Amsterdam, and director of the Digital Interactions Lab. Her research focusses on better understanding how people learn, and on how innovative technologies can best support their learning. She is particularly interested in working with people with disabilities, particularly autism and ADHD, to design technologies which improve their lived experiences.

**Simon S. Hackett,** PhD, is a consultant art psychotherapist in the UK working for Cumbria, Northumberland, Tyne and Wear NHS Foundation Trust and a senior clinical lecturer in applied mental health research based at the Population Health Sciences Institute, Newcastle University. Simon is a Clinical-Academic Allied Health Professional (AHP), having been awarded three National Institute for Health and Care Research (NIHR) Fellowships. Most recently he has been awarded a Health Education England/NIHR Integrated Clinical Academic (ICA) programme Senior Clinical Lectureship Fellowship. This included funding to conduct the SCHEMA Trial: Secure Care Hospital Evaluation of Manualised Interpersonal Art Psychotherapy – a randomised controlled trial.

**Deborah Haythorne,** MA, is an HCPC registered dramatherapist and is co-chief executive of Roundabout, the largest Dramatherapy charity in the UK. Deborah has maintained a clinical caseload working with children, young people and adults, and has developed a special interest in working with adults with a dual diagnosis of learning disability and mental health issues and working with people with a diagnosis of autism. Deborah has co-edited journal articles and other publications which include *Dramatherapy and Autism* (2017) and *Dramatherapy with Children, Young People and Schools* (2012).

**Rainbow Tin Hung Ho,** PhD, BC-DMT, AThR, REAT, RSMT, CGP, CMA, is the associate dean, Faculty of Social Sciences; professor, Department of Social Work and Social Administration; director, Centre on Behavioral Health, and master of Expressive Arts Therapy programme in the University of Hong Kong. She is a board-certified dance movement therapist, a registered expressive arts therapist and somatic movement therapist, a certified group psychotherapist, a movement analyst, and a medical technologist. She is also a registered dance teacher in classical ballet and ballroom dances, and a licensed international dance sport adjudicator. Prof. Ho publishes extensively in refereed journals, scholarly books and encyclopaedia, and has been the principal investigator of many research projects related to mind-body medicine, Creative Arts Therapy, and physical activity for various populations. She received the Research Award (2015, 2019) and the Outstanding Achievement Award (2015) from the American Dance Therapy Association; and received the Research and Development Award from the Australia and New Zealand Arts Therapy Association in 2016.

**Kate Howland,** PhD, is a senior lecturer in Interaction Design at the Department of Informatics at the University of Sussex (UK). A key focus in her work is the design and evaluation of learning environments for children, particularly those that involve embodied interaction. Her research explores how end users can take a more active role in the creation of novel technologies, and places an emphasis on the importance of understanding real-world learning contexts.

**Vicky Karkou,** PhD, is a professor, qualified researcher, educator, teacher and creative psychotherapist (dance movement psychotherapist), having worked with vulnerable children and adults in schools, voluntary organisations and the NHS. She moved to Edge Hill University in 2013, leading the Research Centre for Arts and Wellbeing. In 2014, she was awarded an honorary Doctor of Medicine at Riga Stradins University in recognition of her contribution to the development of arts therapies training in Latvia. She is well-published in national and international journals, and has written and edited books, while also acting as the co-editor for the international journal *Body, Movement and Dance in Psychotherapy,* published by Taylor and Francis. She travels extensively while continuing to supervise masters and PhD studies. She has recently supported the development of a new MSc in Contemporary Creative Approaches to Psychotherapy and Counselling, which received its first cohort in 2019.

**KerryLyn Kercher,** MA, R-DMT, LPCC, is a dance/movement therapist at the Children's Hospital Colorado for patient populations in both the mental health hospital and medical units. Kerrylyn holds a BFA in dance

performance from Shenandoah Conservatory and an MA in dance/
movement therapy and counselling from Drexel University, and is a
Germany Fulbright recipient 2021–2022 under study and research
within the Research Institute for Creative Arts Therapies (RIArT) at
Alanus University in Alfter/Bonn. KerryLyn's creative curiosities include
creative art therapies as treatment modalities for depression, anxiety,
autism, trauma and attachment-related disorders.

**Sabine C. Koch**, MA, BC-DMT, PhD, is psychologist and dance/movement
therapist, professor of dance/movement therapy at SRH University
Heidelberg, and director of the Research Institute for Creative Arts
Therapies (RIArT) at Alanus University in Alfter/Bonn. Sabine's research
areas include Embodiment research, Kestenberg Movement Profiling,
Dance/Movement Therapy and depression, trauma, autism, schizophrenia
and the elderly.

**Jeannie Lewis**, MA, completed her MA Dramatherapy Training at
Roehampton in 2007. Jeannie has worked with a range of different
client groups including children in Sure Start and early years, and
primary and secondary aged children in mainstream and special schools.
She has worked with Specialist Autism Spectrum Condition services and
with Autistic children and young adults in schools, specialist schools and in
private practice. Jeannie has a particular interest in working imaginatively
with young people on the Autistic Spectrum and has published in
the *BADTH Journal* on this subject and contributed a chapter to
*Dramatherapy and Autism* (2017). Jeannie is a creative arts supervisor,
approved by Creative Arts Supervision Training (CAST). She currently
works as a freelance dramatherapist with Roundabout Dramatherapy and
as an employed dramatherapist in schools. She also runs Supervision
groups for MA training courses and works as a clinical supervisor and
therapist in private practice.

**Ryan Matchullis**, PhD, is a registered psychologist and PhD graduate of the
School and Applied Child Psychology Program at the University of
Calgary, Alberta. He has a full-time role with Alberta Health Services
Autism Diagnostic Clinic and Cumulative Risk Diagnostic Clinic, as well
as a private practice with a focus on neurodevelopmental assessment
family supports.

**Daniel Mateos-Moreno**, PhD, was educated in institutions from varied
countries, including the University of Cambridge (UK), Carnegie-Mellon
University (USA) and the University of Malaga (Spain). Daniel holds
degrees in piano, holds degrees from the University of Cambridge in the
UK and from Carnegie Mellon University in Pittsburgh, USA. He is currently

working as an associate professor in music education at the University of Malaga in Spain. Previously, he held the position of Reader in music pedagogy at the University of Karlstad in Sweden. He has taught modules and supervised doctoral dissertations in creative art therapies and has authored works published in *Psychology of Music, Music Education Research*, and *The Arts in Psychotherapy*. He is the happy father of two children, a cat, and a dog, and enjoys composing music and reading about physics.

**Janet Tein Ni Moo**, MSc (King's College London), MA (Goldsmiths University of London), is a PhD candidate at the University of Hong Kong and a registered Dance Movement Psychotherapist (ADMP UK). Since introducing Dance Movement Psychotherapy (DMP) to Malaysia in 2010, she has trained teachers and psychologists at the National Autism Society of Malaysia, and founded Flow Within, a company which collaborates with special needs centres to offer DMP to individuals with autism. In the UK, she has worked as a DMP at several Special Educational Needs and Disabilities (SEND) schools and colleges. She also pioneered the dance programme for the London PE & School Sports Network, for children and adolescents with autism. Currently, she is working on her thesis on autism and DMP under the supervision of Prof. Rainbow Tin Hung Ho, a board-certified dance/movement therapist.

**Nicki Power** is an art therapist, currently undertaking an Allied Health Professions Clinical Doctoral Fellowship with the Queen Mary University of London, awarded by Barts Charity. She is working collaboratively with people with a learning disability, using arts-based methods, to develop and test group art therapy. She was formerly Head of Arts Therapies for Bedfordshire Adult Mental Health & Learning Disability Services, East London NHS Foundation Trust. She is a coordinator of the British Association of Art Therapists: Learning Disability Professional Support Group. She is a member of the editorial board for the *Irish Journal of Creative Arts Therapies: Polyphony*.

**Grazia Ragone** is a doctoral researcher and doctoral tutor at the University of Sussex in Brighton (UK). She completed her first degree in musicology at the Italian University of Pavia and a master's degree in music and art therapy at the University of Tor Vergata in Rome, where she became a practitioner working mainly with autistic children. Subsequently, she moved to the UK where she completed a postgraduate qualification in developmental psychology at the London Metropolitan University and a master's degree in psychological research methods at the University of Sussex, where she is now a PhD candidate in human-computer interaction (HCI). Her research lies at the intersection of computer science and developmental psychology, with a particular interest in HCI for supporting the learning and interactive practices of autistic children. Grazia has been awarded the 1st prize in the Student Research Competition at ASSETS20, from Microsoft Research and the best work-in-progress paper at the Interaction Design for Children Conference (IDC20). Also, she received an official citation from The Massachusetts Senate in 2012 in recognition for dedication and commitment to autism research.

**Emma Ramsden,** PhD, practitioner-researcher and clinical supervisor (HCPC), has more than two decades of experience in the field of Dramatherapy in the UK. She currently leads on a range of research projects including dramatherapists' perception of child agency in collaboration with Professor Phil Jones at UCL's Institute of Education (IOE). Recent publications include the co-authored book *Child Agency and Voice in Therapy: New Ways of Working in the Arts Therapies* (2020) and the chapter "Role Theory and the Role Method of Drama Therapy Explored Through the Case of Peter Pan" in *Current Approaches in Drama Therapy* (2020).

**Grace Thompson,** PhD, is a registered music therapist and associate professor of music therapy at the University of Melbourne. Grace has worked with children, young people and families for over 20 years within the early childhood intervention and special education sector. Within her music therapy practice, Grace developed a collaborative approach to working with families guided by ecological theories and family-centred philosophy. Her PhD investigated outcomes of home-based music therapy sessions with preschool-aged autistic children and their mothers. Grace's research continues to explore the ways music therapists can foster relationships and social connection through accessible music making. Grace is past president of the Australian Music Therapy Association, author of *Goal Processes in Music Therapy Practice*, and co-editor of the book *Music Therapy with Families: Therapeutic Approaches and Theoretical Perspectives*. She is currently editor in chief of the *Nordic Journal of Music Therapy*.

# Preface

*Arts Therapies Research with Persons on the Autism Spectrum: Colourful Hatchlings* is a collection of international research studies from art, music, drama, dance or combined Creative Arts Therapies or Arts Therapies. As a research text, it contributes towards the development and consolidation of effective, scalable approaches for the management and support of the diverse needs of persons on the Autism Spectrum. The three sections of this book capture ways of working with the neurodiverse population across the age span and settings through Creative Arts Therapies delivered in person or digitally. The book presents some of the most recent findings from good quality and rigorously conducted research using diverse methodologies including case studies, arts-based research, clinical trials and interviews to comprehensively represent the views of children, parents, educators, therapists and researchers. As such it offers a comprehensive picture of core aspects of practice, therapeutic trends, research evidence on processes and outcomes across arts therapies for persons on the autism spectrum.

This book will therefore be of interest to arts therapies researchers, practitioners, trainees, special educators and other health care professionals, particularly those who work with neurodiverse clients. By making the work of arts therapists accessible globally, it is expected to open doors for novel possibilities in the lives of people on the autism spectrum.

# Acknowledgements

We are deeply indebted to Marcus Bull for his timely support for proofreading the chapters and offering highly valuable comments. We would like to express our personal appreciation to Rohini Mohan, K G Rajalakshmi, Arnav, Ina and the children from Sarayu Kala Kuteera, Bengaluru for adding more colours, imagination and creativity to this book. This endeavour would not have been possible without Gnanavel who extended his technical support, and shared his honest views with patience to complete this work.

# Foreword

### Do people with Autism feel?

> Loneliness is not the absence of people. Loneliness is the inability to express what matters to you most.
>
> – Carl Jung

This quote is the touchstone of much of our work on Arts and Health at the World Health Organization and speaks to how creativity is more than merely a pathway to health, but an intrinsic part of what it means to be a healthy human. In the context of autism, this quote has a deeper poignancy, as the set of conditions we identify under the umbrella of autism all have one thing in common: the neurological disruption of our ability to express or understand what matters most to each other.

This volume represents a snapshot of the current state of how creative expression can be used in the treatment and management of autism. Each chapter is research-based, and taken altogether, the chapters span 4 continents, over 30 countries, across all of the arts therapies and demographic groups, showing what techniques have been effective, and outlining what areas may profit by future study.

But if autism, in all its forms, has as a common denominator an inability to read emotions, then ironically, it has that attribute in common with academic writing. Taking advantage of the freedom offered me by being the author of a foreword rather than an academic chapter, I intend to briefly counter balance the excellent evidence-based writing in this important volume with, dare I say it, anecdote.

Autism is more common than we would like to think, some say as high as one in a hundred can be placed somewhere on the spectrum. In my own family, there is a cousin who is autistic, and the family for the most part deals with her condition by ignoring it, allowing her to join all functions, but not acknowledging her condition in any overt way. At family gatherings, she would often sit alone with no interaction with the others, under the assumption that simply being together gave her, and her family, some sense of belonging, but with little outward sign of it. At one summer picnic, I overheard one family member muse aloud in front of her "I wonder if she feels anything at all?"

The question of whether a person with autism 'feels' is a bit like the question of Schrödinger's Cat. Studies cited in the July 12, 2016, edition of *Scientific American* in an article by Rebecca Brewer and Jennifer Murphy suggest that only 50% of people living with autism also have alexithymia (inability to read or process emotions). By way of comparison, this is roughly the same rate as clinical depression. The two conditions are distinct, even if they often overlap. This means that without a detailed and accurate diagnostic, when you interact with someone with autism, you have to assume that they can feel emotions and that they can't. Accommodations must be made without assumptions. The creative arts can help those who feel but can't express find that expression. They can also help those who can't feel, and find a level of normalcy and interaction to help them make sense of the world and live a fulfilled life.

A number of years ago, I directed a stage production of Mary Shelly's Frankenstein on the 200th anniversary of the publication of the novel. During the auditions for the creature, I noted that most of the actors were reflexively performing some variation of the lumbering behemoth we have come to be familiar with in screen adaptations over the decades. However, there was one young Zimbabwean man who tried something totally unique. His performance of the creature was almost like a wild dog, totally spontaneous and primal. I asked him during the audition if he was familiar with the story either by watching a film or reading the novel. He said he didn't know the story. He was creating a totally original and pure interpretation, all on instinct.

A week later when I offered him the role, he told me as a disclaimer that he was autistic. He said he would understand if I cast someone else. I asked him what that meant in terms of rehearsals. Would he have difficulty memorizing his lines? He said he didn't know, he hadn't acted in a major stage production before. So we both took the risk together.

In some aspects, his condition actually aided the rehearsal process. His ability to obsessively repeat behaviors came in handy in terms of memorization and establishing blocking. And at other times, it offered challenges. During the scene when he confronts his 'bride', I staged it almost as a mirroring exercise, not unlike the techniques described in Chapter 10 of this volume. The scene wasn't working. He was never actually looking at his bride's face so the text actually did not make any sense. When I asked him to pay attention to the face of the actress playing his bride, he quietly informed me that it is a symptom of his condition. It is very difficult for him to look at faces, which is one of the reasons why people with autism have such a difficult time reading emotions of others, as the eyes and the mouth are often the most obvious transmitters of emotional cues. So I told him that he didn't actually have to look at her face, but that he should try to, and feel the difficulty of that moment authentically. The result was an absolutely riveting and heartbreaking scene.

During the performances, there was no public mention of his neurological condition. The performance built upon his unique characteristics and skills while compensating for his deficits. The result was that the audience felt the same thrill I felt during the audition. This was something totally unique and authentic, even if we had no idea why.

During the intermission of one of the performances, his doctor approached me, introduced himself and asked if I was the director. He then proceeded to tell me that after years under his care, in the few short weeks of the rehearsal process, this young man for the first time began to share his enthusiasm with his family, began to bridle at things being done for him, insisting that he do them himself, and that week hit a major milestone in his life. He moved out of his mother's home to his own apartment. But most significantly, he expressed happiness and pride. The doctor told me that he has no idea what I had done in rehearsals to afford this change, but whatever it was it worked. I told him I did nothing, except observed, listened, and helped him unlock his own instincts and choices, the same way I would with any actor.

When asking permission to use the personal story above, I received the following response which due to its charm, I am sharing in its entirety.

I have read through the draft and you have my permission to use it. Also, I would like to add a few words about my experience working with you on Frankenstein: This experience helped me to come out of my shell. It helped me memorize my lines, understand my character and create my bond with my fellow actors and actresses. Acting is my passion and I realized that when I started working with Chris because he understood me. I appreciate everything that Chris has done for me. Hopefully I can continue my passion for acting. Finally, I prefer to be named so you also have my permission.
(Tinashe, 20.2.2023)

Like our definition of Health, the WHO definition of Mental Health is asset not deficit-based. Mental Health is not merely the alleviation of conditions, symptoms or disabilities. To gauge one's Mental Health, you must ask yourselves the questions 'can I cope with the everyday stress of life?' 'Can I practice my abilities to their highest individual potential?' 'Am I productive?' 'Do I participate in a community?' And dare I add, 'can I find moments of joy?' If the answers to these questions are yes, then you have mental health regardless of what diagnosable conditions you may or may not have.

The creative arts may indeed reduce symptoms of mental disorders such as autism in some measurable aspect. But that is not their real value. They allow us to reconnect with ourselves, each other and the world around us in a way that is personally authentic and communally beneficial. The arts do not need to cure to be able to heal. They help us curate our lives.

Christopher Bailey
February 19, 2023
Arts and Health Lead
World Health Organization

# Introduction

## Steering the Road Map of Arts Therapies Research with Persons on the Autism Spectrum

*Supritha Aithal and Vicky Karkou*

Individual differences among human beings are probably as infinite as the colours in the electromagnetic spectrum. However, our human vision is limited, allowing us to see only particular shades, which we can group and name, assigning some as primary colours. Similarly, our perceptions of similarities and differences among individuals lead us to categorise people with identities and associated labels. One such category is the autism spectrum, a label that refers to approximately one in one hundred people across the globe with perceived similarities in social, communication and behavioural patterns (Zeidan et al., 2022).

Over the past century, our understanding and perception of autism have evolved, and it continues to change. Many differences in the terminologies can be noticed starting from Kanner (1943), who first documented his clinical observations of unusual and stereotypical behavioural patterns, to the latest revisions of diagnostic manuals such as (i) the International Classification of Diseases (ICD), produced by the World Health Organization (WHO) to classify and codify diseases and disorders of all kinds globally, and (ii) the Diagnostic and Statistical Manual of Mental Disorders (*DSM*), by the American Psychiatric Association (Tyrer et al., 2014). Previously, separate diagnoses of childhood autism, Asperger's syndrome, Rett's Syndrome, Childhood Disintegrative Disorder (CDD) and Pervasive Developmental Disorder Not Otherwise Specified (PDD-NOS) were in use. Currently, both classification systems (*DSM-5* and ICD-11) have put all these into a single category of Autism Spectrum Disorder (ASD); they define ASD as a neurodevelopmental disorder identified by a persistent deficit in social communication and interaction, with restricted, repetitive patterns of behaviour (APA, 2013; Regier et al., 2013; First et al., 2021). This medical or diagnostic model depends upon external observations of behavioural patterns and offers a deficit-based understanding.

In such diagnostic models, symptoms and characteristics are categorised from the perspectives of people who have not lived the lives of people with

DOI: 10.4324/9781003201656-1

ASD. By contrast, the self-advocacy-informed neurodiversity movement offers an internal view of the autism spectrum and provides a voice for autistic people. The neurodiversity movement acknowledges differences in how people experience the world. It considers that one person's ability to communicate and process information will differ from the typical trend, and states that autism spectrum is simply one such form of neurodivergence (Farmer, Ciaunica and Hamilton, 2018). Autistic people display a wide range of abilities; while their behaviour may appear different from those without autism they can be accepted in their social contexts as they are (Autism and Neurodiversity, 2019). This movement criticises the norm-centric notion that ASDs are pathological medical conditions in need of diagnosis, normalisation and cure (Straus, 2014).

The deficit model identifies interventions aiming towards outcomes that potentially modify behaviours perceived as challenging, behaviours that typically do not fit within societal norms. Authors who align with the diagnostic manual conventions use people-first language, such as 'child/adult with ASD', to express that the condition is not the most important or defining characteristic of the person. However, the self-advocates prefer to be addressed as 'autistic individuals', making the point that autism is an integral part of their identity and not something that needs to be treated. The principles of this neurodiversity paradigm state that there is no valid way to claim a normal or healthy brain, nor one right way of neurocognitive processing; rather, there are infinite ways of neurocognitive processing and people with autism have their own unique ways. Just like any other form of diversity in society, such as skin colour, ethnicity or language, neurodiversity is also subject to social dynamics including dynamics of power and oppression (Walker, 2021). The neurodiversity movement identifies the need for change in society, with a focus on the quality of life, resilience and strengths (Szatmari, 2018; Turry, 2018), while the deficit model claims that the behavioural patterns of the individual need modification. Both models, although taking different approaches, aim toward social integration and better functioning. In this book, we acknowledge both paradigms, appreciate the differences in the use of language and settings and offer creative ways of finding a middle ground. We believe that shades from contrasting ends of the spectrum can meet and blend to create a wide-ranging palette of colours for supporting each other through arts therapies/ creative arts therapies.

Arts therapies/Creative arts therapies is a collective term that refers to the disciplines of art therapy/psychotherapy, music therapy, dramatherapy and dance movement therapy/psychotherapy, all of which use artistic media for therapeutic interaction, engagement and eventually therapeutic change (Karkou and Sanderson, 2006). Although there are crossovers and similarities, they are also distinct in terms of history, artistic preferences and models of practice across different cultural settings. All these disciplines, however, are held together by common factors such as art-making processes, creativity, playfulness, imagery, symbolism, metaphor, and non verbal communication. In all cases, the client-therapist relationship is placed at the heart of the process.

Arts therapies have advanced over the years, not only addressing the diverse needs of people on the autism spectrum and their families but also playing a key role in raising awareness in society (Sharda et al., 2018; Aithal et al., 2021b). There are increasing numbers of arts therapists working with this client population across age, severity and spectrum of needs in various settings. In a survey of practitioners by Karkou and Sanderson (2006), 30% of arts therapists in the UK reported that they were working with clients experiencing learning, multiple or physical/sensory difficulties; autism was likely within one of these three categories. An updated survey some years later (Zubala et al., 2013; Zubala and Karkou, 2015) showed that this trend persisted. Particularly, the popular trend appeared to be working in schools and special schools with music therapists and dance movement psychotherapists (Karkou, 2010). Similarly, as per the survey results of Carr et al. (2017), music therapists most frequently work with children who have developmental and behavioural challenges. Some individuals on the autism spectrum display particular artistic abilities. In music, for example, there are people with autism who show advanced abilities to recognise pitch and timbre and/or who have excellent musical memory and high levels of aptitude to process melodic and rhythmic intricacies (Fancourt and Finn, 2019). Although extraordinary artistic skills are not necessary to take part in arts therapies, an inclination and interest to engage with the artistic medium do support the use of arts therapies. In particular, the processes that occur within artistic interaction may reduce barriers to communication and enable human connection without words. Using the arts as a medium for accessing pre-verbal experiences is seen to be more helpful for engaging emotionally on a relationship-oriented level than verbal interaction which requires a predominant cognitive understanding (Geretsegger et al., 2014).

Although there is an upward trend in the growth of quantitative, qualitative, arts-based and mixed-methods research approaches in arts therapies, research in the field presents only a fragmented picture of the potential contribution of arts therapies for this client group. A review of ten studies in music therapy, for example, has demonstrated low to moderate quality evidence of improvement in social interaction, communication, initiating behaviour, social-emotional reciprocity and quality of relationship in persons on the autism spectrum (Geretsegger et al., 2014). Similarly, recent systematic reviews from dance movement therapy (Aithal et al., 2021a), dramatherapy (Bololia et al., 2022) and art therapy (Schweizer et al., 2014) also offer insights on the evidence currently available for this client population. However, in most cases, the evidence relies on small sample sizes and measurement tools that are not well established, limiting the generalisability of the results.

Differences in perception of the autism spectrum are also reflected in the choice of research designs and approaches. For example, the Trial of Improvisational Music Therapy's Effectiveness for Children with Autism (TIME-A) Music Therapy project (Geretsegger et al., 2012) and Toward an

Embodied Science of Intersubjectivity (TESIS), a dance movement therapy project (Mastrominico et al., 2018) that used Randomised Control Trial designs, found no beneficial effects for symptom reduction and improvement of empathy respectively. Contrastingly, there are many qualitative accounts indicating that therapeutic changes can happen (Adler, 1970; Low et al., 2022). As a result, in this book, diverse methodologies – qualitative, quantitative, arts-based and mixed methodologies – are included, offering a comprehensive picture of practice, therapeutic trends, and research evidence on processes and outcomes across arts therapies for persons on the autism spectrum.

The varying needs of this client population are so complex that therapists continue to explore new ways of working. However, more research is needed (Aithal et al., 2021a) to identify and document the most effective methods, techniques and approaches. Our book aims to respond to this need by bringing together international research studies from art, music, drama, dance or movement and combined creative arts therapies, as part of the International Research in the arts therapies series. In recognition of the diverse needs of people with autism and the creative character of arts therapies, the book is sub-titled *Colourful Hatchlings*. As artistically depicted in Figure 0.1, we will present and discuss empirical evidence that sheds light on ways of supporting the wellbeing of persons on the autism spectrum and their families across the lifespan, representing different contexts of work, different configurations and diverse types of services.

This book contains 14 research-based chapters with contributions from 31 authors from around the world, including a variety of research outcomes, therapeutic processes and critiques both of existing practice and research methodologies. The contributors, from the UK, the USA, Canada, the Netherlands, Germany, Spain, Greece, Hong Kong, Singapore and Australia have presented research studies spreading across the age span, settings and services currently available in their contexts for people on the autism spectrum. The chapters are rich with descriptions of different therapeutic approaches from varying philosophical stances. The authors bring in multiple perspectives, weaving their expertise as practitioners and researchers with service users and caregivers. This collective effort of interdisciplinary research showcases the extent of evidence-based practice from around the world.

The chapters are assembled in three parts. The first part, Little Hatchlings, consists of six chapters focusing on arts therapies research with children on the autism spectrum and their families, and an artistic depiction of this can be seen in Figure 0.2. The second part, Blooming Hatchlings, comprises of five chapters exploring research with young people and adults on the autism spectrum (see also Figure 0.3). These two sections pertain to a specific discipline with arts therapies. However, the last part, Coming Together with Hatchlings, contains five chapters integrating combinations and connections across different conditions, timeframes, technology, disciplines and professions for the differing developmental needs of the client group (Figure 0.4). Overall, the chapters

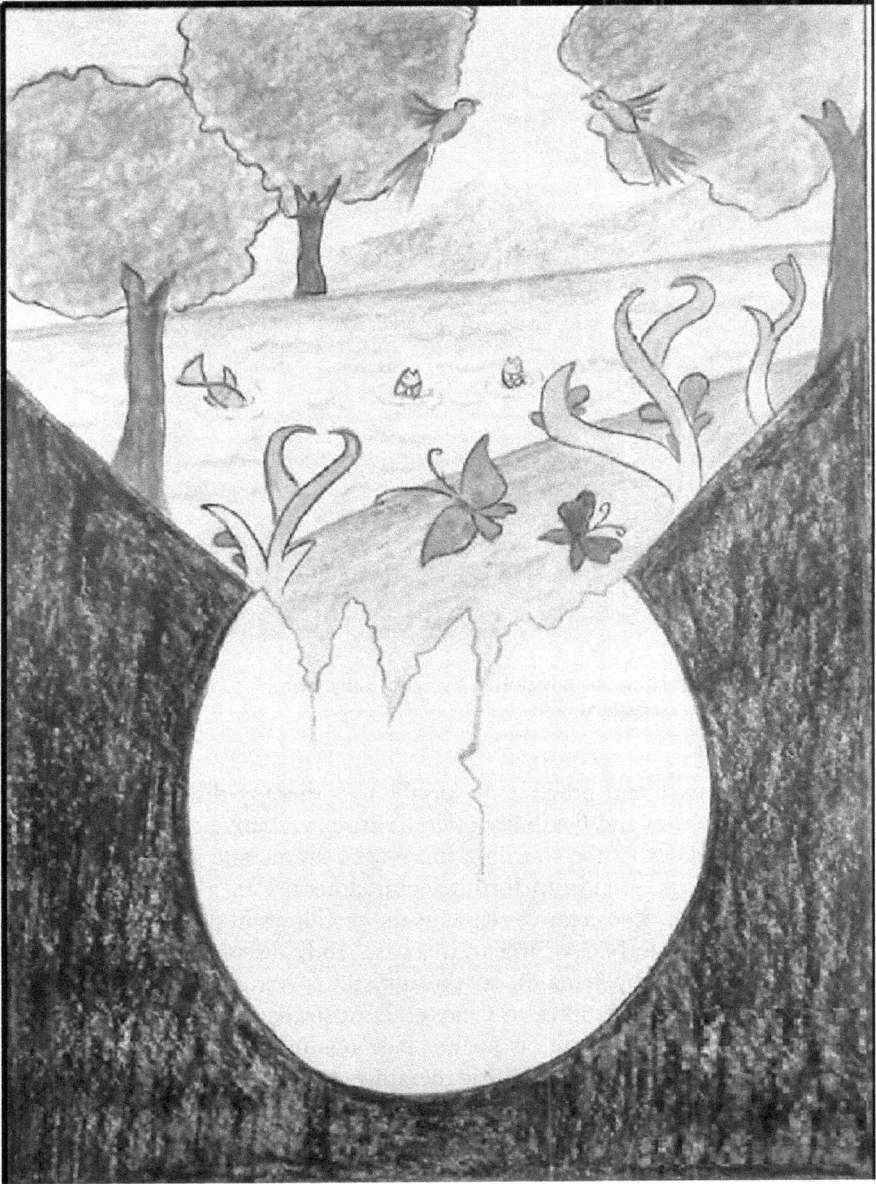

*Figure 0.1* Colourful hatchlings as envisioned by Apoorva Chakraverthy N. (14 years), Sarayu Kala Kuteera, Bengaluru

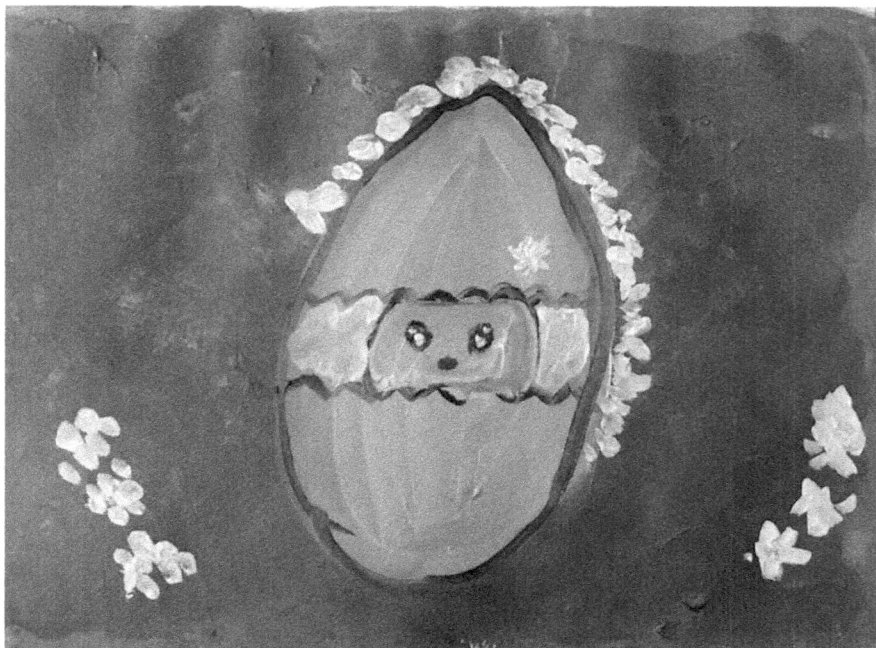

*Figure 0.2* Little hatchlings as envisioned by Diya Bijoy Nambiar (14 years), Sarayu Kala Kuteera, Bengaluru

explore the impact and practice of specific arts therapy discipline as well as highlight the fluidity and flexibility offered through creative connections.

Chapter 1 relates to the touching journey of an autistic girl exploring and finding meaning in friendship through dramatherapy in a UK-based special educational setting. The creative elements on hatchlings in this chapter inspired the title of this book. Nicky Dyer in this case study discusses the unique difficulties encountered by females on the autistic spectrum trying to navigate meaningful social interactions. In Chapter 2, Australian music therapist Grace Thompson reevaluates results from her past qualitative research studies and proposes a framework for how music therapists can support parents to support their children by working with family-centred principles. This chapter is strongly informed by the neurodiversity movement and advocates for the voice of lived experience, social justice and social change. The next chapter is a qualitative study by an international team, Andrea Gleason, Christina Devereaux and Ryan Matchullis, that offers an educators' view of the role of dance movement therapy to support children on the autism spectrum in Canadian early intervention classrooms. The results highlight the different therapeutic factors of DMT and explain how adopting person-centred principles can let children have a 'movement voice'. Chapter 4 focuses on the Sensory-

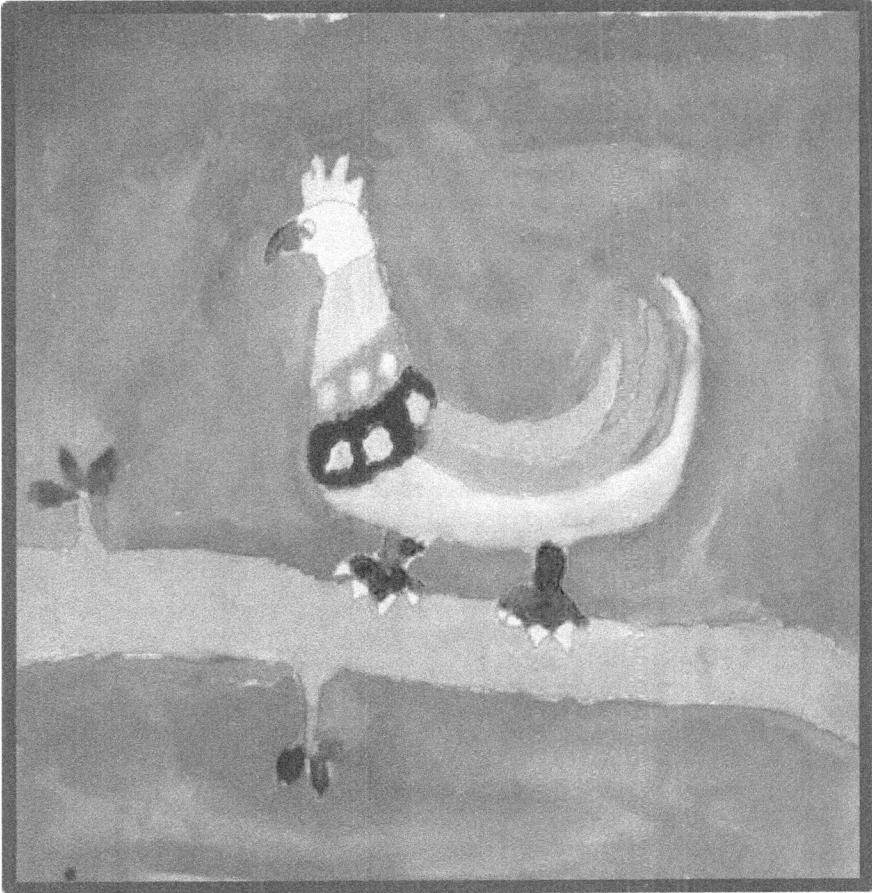

*Figure 0.3* Blooming hatchling (in isolation) as envisioned by Arnav Bhamati Kothari (11 years), Mysuru

Based Relational Art Therapy Approach (S-BRATA) developed by Huma Durrani through her research work in Singapore. Using three case vignettes, the chapter offers suggestions and practical tips for practitioners to apply in their practice. Chapter 5 is from the Roundabout dramatherapy company in the UK. Emma Ramsden and the Roundabout team in this qualitative study explore a specific routine evaluation and research tool to give voice to the children on their experience of being in a dramatherapy group. In the final chapter of part 1, Laura Blauth introduces a newly developed assessment tool to evaluate the quality of relationship. She discusses its use within the music therapy sessions and presents case vignettes, illustrating the resilience-informed framework to understand the characteristics of the work and processes of therapeutic change.

Chapters 7–10 are dedicated to research on arts therapies with young people and adults on the autism spectrum. This section begins with a chapter from a dance movement therapy study by Sabine Koch and Kerry Lyn Kercher from Germany and the USA, respectively. Through the secondary reflexive research of existing empirical evidence on mirroring, they provide a theoretical frame to Mirroring Intervention Protocol (MIP) and raise key questions for further research on the impact of mirroring techniques on empathy and attachment patterns of adults on the autism spectrum. In Chapter 8, Simon Hackett, an art therapist from the UK, describes an in-depth single case study from a larger trial. This chapter provides a detailed explanation of the process and impact of an interpersonal art psychotherapy approach for an adult on the autism spectrum within secure care. Chapter 9 is on adolescents participating in a dramatherapy intervention from a study conducted in Greece. Loukia Bololia examines themes that emerged from interviews with parents on the impact of dramatherapy on the participants. In the last chapter of this section, Daniel Mateos-Moreno and Lidia Atencia-Doña from Spain utilise the connection between dance and music to explore

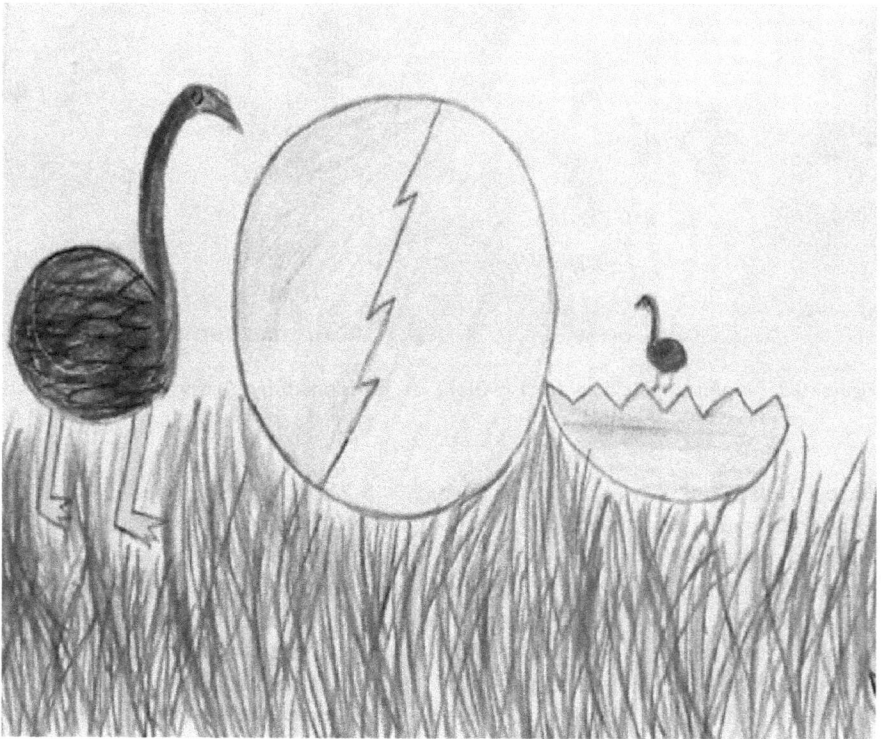

*Figure 0.4* Coming together with hatchlings as envisioned by Aprameya S. Kaniyar (14 years) Sarayu Kala Kuteera, Bengaluru

the impact of combined dance movement and music therapy for adults on the autism spectrum.

The final section, Chapters 11–14, brings out unique connections and combinations of arts therapies research with persons on the autism spectrum. In Chapter 11, Janet Tein Ni Moo and Rainbow Tin Hung Ho, from Hong Kong, connect with dance movement therapists around the world to understand the use of tele-dance movement therapy for children and adolescents on the autism spectrum during the recent COVID-19 pandemic. Similarly, connections with technology and music therapy and interdisciplinarity are demonstrated through narrative and reflective research in Chapter 12 by Grazia Ragone with her international research team. This chapter traces the journey of a music therapist with training in Human-Computer Interaction (HCI) prototyping a digital music therapy approach with autistic children. The next chapter focuses on nonverbal autistic children and the importance of attunement. Jeannie Lewis, a dramatherapist from the UK, demonstrates how different professionals working with a common client population come together to find different ways of meeting the clients' needs. Finally, in the last chapter, Nicki Power, an art therapist and researcher from the UK, narrates the story of a pioneer art therapist's (Roger Arguile) work with long-term client Marshall Bourne and his mother Kerry Bourne. They all reconnect three years after ending therapy to reflect on their past experiences and to explore their views on the therapeutic factors, therapeutic alliances and long-term benefits of art therapy. Celebrated in this chapter is the power of genuine connections through the medium of art, making a real difference to ways of being.

In summary, by looking at arts therapies research in this area, this book intends to contribute to the development and consolidation of effective, scalable approaches for the management and support of the diverse needs of persons on the autism spectrum and their caregivers. This may, in turn, have an impact on societal perceptions about autism, creating policies and making arts therapies accessible to a wider range of client population globally and opening doors for novel possibilities in the Lives of people on the autism spectrum.

## References

Adler, J. (1970). *Looking For Me*. Extension Media Center. University of CA, Berkeley.

Aithal, S., Moula, Z., Karkou, V., Karaminis, T., Powell, J. and Makris, S. (2021a) 'A systematic review of the contribution of dance movement psychotherapy towards the well-being of children with autism spectrum disorders', *Frontiers in Psychology*, 12, p. 719673. Available at: 10.3389/fpsyg.2021.719673.

Aithal, S., Karkou, V., Makris, S., Karaminis, T. and Powell, J. (2021b) 'Impact of dance movement psychotherapy on the wellbeing of caregivers of children with autism spectrum disorder', *Public Health*, 200, pp. 109–115. Available at: 10.101 6/j.puhe.2021.09.018.

American Psychiatric Association (2013) *Diagnostic and statistical manual of mental disorders 5 Ed DSM-5*. 5th edition. Washington, D.C.: CBS.

Autism and Neurodiversity (2019) Available at: https://www.sendgateway.org.uk/ download.neurodiversity-information-leaflet_1.html (Accessed 18 January 2020).

Bololia, L., Williams, J.M., Goodall, K. and Macmahon, K. (2022) 'Dramatherapy for children and adolescents with autism spectrum disorder: A systematic integrative review', *Arts in Psychotherapy*, 80, p. 101918. Available at: 10.1016/ j.aip.2022.101918.

Carr, C.E., Tsiris, G. and Swijghuisen Reigersberg, M. (2017) 'Understanding the present, re-visioning the future: An initial mapping of music therapists in the United Kingdom', *British Journal of Music Therapy*, 31(2), pp. 68–85. Available at: 10.1177/1359457517728379.

Fancourt, D. and Finn, S. (2019) *What is the evidence on the role of the arts in improving health and well-being? A scoping review.* Copenhagen: WHO Regional Office for Europe (WHO Health Evidence Network Synthesis Reports. Available at: http://www.ncbi.nlm.nih.gov/books/NBK553773/ (Accessed 4 October 2022).

Farmer, H., Ciaunica, A. and de C. Hamilton, A.F. (2018) 'The functions of imitative behaviour in humans', *Mind & Language*, 33, pp. 378–396. Available at: 10.1111/ mila.12189.

First, M.B., Gaebel, W., Maj, M., Stein, D.J., Kogan, C.S., Saunders, J.B., Poznyak, V.B., Gureje, O., Lewis-Fernández, R., Maercker, A., Brewin, C.R., Cloitre, M., Claudino, A., Pike, K.M., Baird, G., Skuse, D., Krueger, R.B., Briken, P., Burke, J.D., Lochman, J.E., Evans, S.C., Woods, D.W. and Reed, G.M. (2021) 'An organization- and category-level comparison of diagnostic requirements for mental disorders in ICD-11 and DSM-5', *World Psychiatry*, 20(1), pp. 34–51. Available at: 10.1002/wps.20825.

Geretsegger, M., Elefant, C., Mössler, K.A. and Gold, C. (2014) 'Music therapy for people with autism spectrum disorder', *The Cochrane Database of Systematic Reviews*, (6), p. CD004381. Available at: 10.1002/14651858.CD004381.pub3.

Geretsegger, M., Holck, U. and Gold, C. (2012) 'Randomised controlled trial of improvisational music therapy's effectiveness for children with autism spectrum disorders (TIME-A): Study protocol', *BMC Pediatrics*, 12, p. 2. Available at: 10.11 86/1471-2431-12-2.

Kanner, L. (1943) 'Autistic disturbances of affective contact', *Nervous Child*, 2, pp. 217–250.

Karkou, V. and Sanderson, P. (2006) *Arts therapies: A research based map of the field, arts therapies.* Available at: 10.1016/B978-0-443-07256-7.X5001-3.

Karkou V. (2010) 'Introduction', in V. Karkou (ed.) *Arts Therapies in Schools: Research and Practice*. London: Jessica Kingsley, pp 9–23.

Low, M.Y., McFerran, K.S., Viega, M., Carroll-Scott, A., McGhee Hassrick, E., and Bradt, J. (2022) Exploring the lived experiences of young autistic adults in Nordoff-Robbins music therapy: An interpretative phenomenological analysis. *Nordic Journal of Music Therapy*, pp. 1–24.

Mastrominico, A., Fuchs, T., Manders, E., Steffinger, L., Hirjak, D., Sieber, M., Thomas, E., Holzinger, A., Konrad, A., Bopp, N. and Koch, S.C. (2018) 'Effects of dance movement therapy on adult patients with autism spectrum disorder: A randomized controlled trial', *Behavioral Sciences (Basel, Switzerland)*, 8(7), p. E61. Available at: 10.3390/bs8070061.

Regier, D.A., Kuhl, E.A. and Kupfer, D.J. (2013) 'The DSM-5: Classification and criteria changes', *World Psychiatry*, 12(2), pp. 92–98. Available at: 10.1002/wps.2 0050.

Schweizer, C., Knorth, E.J. and Spreen, M. (2014) 'Art therapy with children with autism spectrum disorders: A review of clinical case descriptions on "what works"', *The Arts in Psychotherapy*, 41, pp. 577–593. Available at: 10.1016/j.aip.2014.10.009.

Sharda, M., Tuerk, C., Chowdhury, R., Jamey, K., Foster, N., Custo-Blanch, M., Tan, M., Nadig, A. and Hyde, K. (2018) 'Music improves social communication and auditory–motor connectivity in children with autism', *Translational Psychiatry*, 8(1), pp. 1–13. Available at: 10.1038/s41398-018-0287-3.

Straus, J. (2014) 'Music therapy and autism: A view from disability studies', *Voices: A World Forum for Music Therapy*, 14(3). Available at: 10.15845/voices.v14i3.785.

Szatmari, P. (2018) 'Risk and resilience in autism spectrum disorder: A missed translational opportunity?', *Developmental Medicine & Child Neurology*, 60(3), pp. 225–229. Available at: 10.1111/dmcn.13588.

Turry, A. (2018) 'Response to effects of improvisational music therapy vs. enhanced standard care on symptom severity among children with autism spectrum disorder: The TIME-A randomized clinical trial', *Nordic Journal of Music Therapy*, 27(1), pp. 87–89. Available at: 10.1080/08098131.2017.1394902.

Tyrer, P. (2014) 'A comparison of DSM and ICD classifications of mental disorder', *Advances in Psychiatric Treatment*, 20(4), pp. 280–285. Available at: 10.1192/apt.bp.113.011296.

Walker, N. (2021) 'What is neurodiversity', Available at: https://www.liebertpub.com/doi/10.1089/aut.2020.29014.njw.

Zeidan, J., Fombonne, E., Scorah, J., Ibrahim, A., Durkin, M.S., Saxena, S., Yusuf, A., Shih, A. and Elsabbagh, M. (2022) 'Global prevalence of autism: A systematic review update', *Autism Research: Official Journal of the International Society for Autism Research*, 15(5), pp. 778–790. Available at: 10.1002/aur.2696.

Zubala, A. and Karkou, V. (2015) 'Dance movement psychotherapy practice in the UK: Findings from the arts therapies survey 2011' body, movement and dance in psychotherapy', 10(1), pp. 21–38. 10.1080/17432979.2014.920918

Zubala, A., Karkou V., MacIntyre D. and Gleeson N. (2013) 'Description of arts therapies practice with adults suffering from depression in the UK: Quantitative results from the nationwide survey', *The Arts in Psychotherapy*, 40(5), pp. 458–464 10.1016/j.aip.2014.10.005.

# Part I

# Little Hatchlings – Arts Therapies with Children on the Autism Spectrum and Their Families

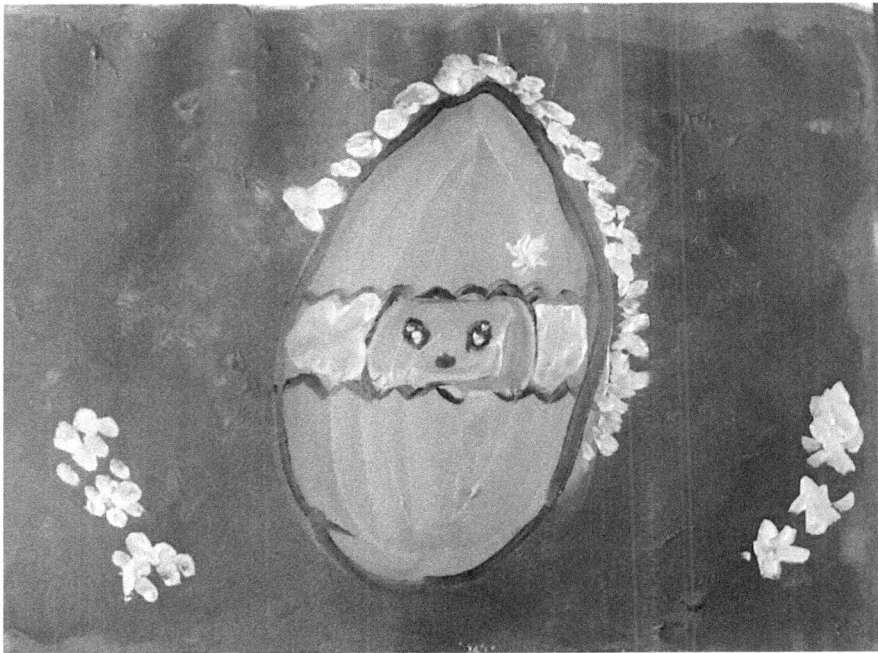

Chapter 1

# Looking After the Hatchlings
## Exploring the Reciprocal Nature of Friendship with an Autistic Girl Through Dramatherapy

*Nicky Dyer*

## Introduction

In Kathryn Erskine's touching and deeply perceptive book *Mockingbird* (2010), we meet protagonist Caitlin – an autistic teenage girl. She just wants to 'fit in' with her peer group and not be vilified for her apparent 'oddities'. As she begins to acquire an appreciation of friendship skills, Caitlin declares in angst that it is not easy for anyone to understand people and find friends.

There is a general view that autistic individuals do not want, are not able or do not feel inclined to participate in social relationships (Daniel and Billingsley, 2010; NICE, 2011). There is even a suggestion that they are content with their own company. In my experience of working with this client group, this is certainly not the case at all. They crave friendship and are extremely unhappy not to have companions. Their anguish seems to stem from the fact that they are unclear as to how to make the necessary or appropriate approaches to others. They seem to find it difficult to unpick other people's thoughts that may differ from their own, listen to the nuances of language or read the signals of expected behaviour (Happe and Frith, 1995). They may need significantly more time to integrate these vital skills to achieve successful relationships than their neurotypical peers (Hughes, 2017).

### The Art of Friendship

Friendship is defined as the affiliative formation of social or emotional bonds with others or the desire to do so which is exclusive of sex or family (Bukowski, Newcomb and Hartup, 1996). It is the single most important factor in influencing our health, wellbeing and happiness (Conn 2014). For stable social interaction to take place, humans need to acquire the abilities of empathy, emotional literacy and reciprocity (Bauminger, Shulman and Agam, 2003).

Research into how typically developing (TD) male and female friendships mature suggests that boys participate in activities alongside each other such as football or sport enabling the inclusion of the autistic individual (Hiller, Young and Weber, 2014). Male interests – for example computer games – help

DOI: 10.4324/9781003201656-3

with this and evolve with age. Female activities thrive on communication and emotional connection. Engagement in female interests does not always translate into teenage life especially if the activities are seen as immature which can lead to bullying and social isolation (Dean, Harwood and Kasari, 2017). This can be mentally overwhelming for autistic girls who are puzzling out the complexities of mindful interaction and results in breakdowns. An emergence of literature documenting autistic female experiences around social integration informs our ongoing awareness of its associated qualities and difficulties (Eaton, 2017).

### The Autistic Female – 'Masking' and 'Camouflaging'

For years, autism has been seen as primarily a male condition (Whitlock et al., 2020). We are now acknowledging that the ratio of girls/women diagnosed on the autistic spectrum is much higher that at first envisaged (Roth et al., 2010). Recorded ratios for males with a diagnosis of autism have stood at 4:10; it has been 10:1 for females, but now this figure is considered to be nearer 6:10 with the probability that it is equal to that of males. One explanation for these revised ratios is that the female phenotype presentation of autism differs from that in males (Tierney et al., 2016).

Autism in males can present with significant behavioural issues, while females seem more proficient in 'masking' or 'camouflaging' their difficulties and copying expected social behaviour by watchfully observing others (Gould and Ashton-Smith, 2011; Milner et al., 2019). The use of 'camouflaging' – an autistic adaptive mechanism (Hull et al., 2017; Bargiela, 2019) makes it possible for females to blend in with their peers and helps them to avoid being bullied or abused (Attwood and Garnett, 2022). Masking requires control and this can prove extraordinarily exhausting leading to bouts of extreme outbursts at home (Moyse and Porter, 2015).

This masking mechanism may explain why females are frequently over-looked or ignored in a diagnosis for autism. Traits such as anxiety, depression, self-harm, eating disorders or obsessive compulsive disorder (OCD) may obscure and override the autism (Dix, 2016). An enriched and deeper understanding of the autistic female perspective is emerging through first-hand accounts which emphasise this fact (Hendrickx, 2015; Bullivant, 2018; May, 2019).

In a documentary about Greta Thurnberg, the Swedish environmental activist (Nessen and Grossman, 2020), it is put to her in an interview that she suffers from autism. In a gentle and measured response, Thurnberg articulates that she would not say she was suffering from it – she just has it. She attributes autism as being the essential force that has enabled her to be able to take on the campaigning in a singularly minded and focussed way - one where she is able to think outside the box. However, as Thurnberg's family testify, there were major struggles before obtaining the diagnosis in 2016.

These included an eating disorder and selective mutism that obscured her autism. Severe depression triggered a critical health crisis before her eventual intense public presence on the world stage (Rourke, 2019).

Hannah Gadsby the Australian comedian asserts that she may have appeared very good at being social but it was an incredibly exhausting process for her. She found her autism diagnosis in 2016 a relief and it helped to put her lived experience into perspective. The diagnosis helped her to create the show 'Nanette' (Bruzzese et al., 2018) in which she presented her personal narrative of growing up with autism and knowing that she was gay. 'Nanette' is by turns hilarious and acutely painful to view and it may have been Gadsby's intention to not only to be heard but understood by people in the hope that there will be changes in society's attitudes.

Her subsequent autobiography – Ten Steps to Nanette – a Memoir Situation (2022) chronicles in even greater depth her immense struggles in achieving the desired balance in her personal life and the joy that she felt when this happened. My aim in offering these high-profile examples is to highlight the complexities around identifying autism in females.

## Study Approach

This chapter aims to answer how dramatherapy supported an autistic girl to explore friendships. Through the case study research approach, I intend to generate an in-depth and multi-faceted understanding of the therapeutic process that facilitated an eight-year-old autistic girl, who I have named Millie (not her real name), to find her way to develop friendship. This is a case study based on detailed process notes written by the therapist accompanied by illustrations and photographs. Permission was sought for this research and all details have been anonymised with any identifying details and names being omitted or changed to protect individuals and institutions.

This intervention took place over the course of an academic year in an English mainstream primary school. To enable each child to achieve their full potential, the school adopted a holistic approach to individual needs. Specific interventions were offered for this purpose including dramatherapy. There was excellent communication between school staff and those delivering these interventions, and this meant pupils progressed well and flourished. I worked in close collaboration with Millie and her family (including her sibling who was also diagnosed with autism) for over four years.

### Case Study

*Millie's life had been in considerable upheaval in the year leading up to this intervention. Her mother had had to deal with a cancer diagnosis and subsequent treatment. Millie's close-knit family were precipitated into childcare challenges, but they worked together to maintain a stable environment for*

*Millie and her sibling. Following the welcome news that her mother's cancer was in remission, Millie began to enjoy life on a more even keel.*

*Millie was diagnosed with autism when seven years old. In relation to DSM-5criteria (APA, 2013), Millie displayed deficits in social-emotional reciprocity with an absence of normal back-and-forth conversation. She found it challenging to develop, maintain and understand relationships and had difficulties in adjusting her behaviour to suit various social contexts (Autism Speaks, 2021). Millie had a real zest for life, her natural exuberance bursting out of her and she was full of imaginative and creative ideas. She longed to consolidate friendships and be part of a group. However, she did not entirely understand how to go about this despite closely observing others (Attwood, 2007). She would become anxious, frustrated and then incredibly exhausted if others did not follow the perceived 'code' that she had worked out. At times meltdowns would ensue which exacerbated her fatigue. The support staff around her were sensitive to this and would diffuse these allowing her space and time to relax and digest what she needed to do next.*

*In Year 4, she was referred for dramatherapy. The emphasis was on the need for Millie to experience a creative outlet to move and express herself freely. During the process, the hope was that she would be able to explore her feelings and practice social and behavioural skills in a safe environment. The referral was made in collaboration with Millie, and she had full autonomy over what happened in the space.*

## Findings

### *The First Phase of Work – We Reflect on What Friendship Is*

When Millie first arrived in the dramatherapy space, she was just bursting with excitement and flitted from activity to activity like a butterfly in a garden of flowers. During this period of settling, I discovered that her main interests were cats, 'My Little Ponies', and Pokémon. The first significant moment of the intervention came when, finding a figure of Bambi in the toy-box, Millie played out the Bambi story (Disney and Hand, 1942). He had lost his mummy and asked the adult deer (the therapist in role) if he had seen her. Bambi said that there had been some hunters around. Was this the reason that Bambi's mum had disappeared? We searched carefully all around the forest (room) but couldn't find Bambi's mum anywhere.

It seemed that she was playing out the scenario of her mother's illness and the fears that she had of her mum dying. This was a poignant moment which I was aware needed to be handled sensitively. I held my breath because I was delighted that Millie was sharing this through the metaphor of the Bambi story. At the same time, I did not want her to become anxious and suddenly 'cut off' from exploring this moment. She had never voiced her thoughts to anyone on how she had been feeling about the illness or indeed the unspoken spectre of possible death that had loomed over the family. I now detected that she seemed comfortable enough to explore this and it helped her to move onto to other work.

In assessing where she was in her development of friendships, I invited her to create a six-part story. This was based on the methodology of Lahad (1992). However, I find Gersie's story structure (1990, 1991) citied by Meldrum (1994) as more 'flexible' to use (See Table 1.1).

*Millie's Story*

The story's simplicity belied the fact that its core was crucial to defining Millie's friendship issues. The story seemed to be portraying a relationship that she had with two other friends in the class. The characters appeared to be different aspects of herself with Boa displaying jealously of other people's friendship and lacking the understanding of knowing how to 'get in' to make a lasting friendship (Figure 1.1). It was this 'getting in' that Millie struggled to negotiate. During this story making, we were able to reflect on friends and friendships and what they mean in general and to us personally. She seemed to know all the right things that you must do to be friends but lacked the understanding of how to put this into practice. She seemed to understand what it is that you should not do to your friends such as being so truthful that it hurts them emotionally or being physically aggressive instead of using words when working issues out. However, she did not have the strategies to work out the alternatives (Figure 1.2).

In our next session we reflected on this, finding out what was good about having friends and writing down words and phrases to illustrate the point. Millie told me that you could talk, laugh, cry, play games together, enjoy picnics, share jokes and sometimes be mischievous as well as being honest with each other. Then we discovered what friends do not do to each other which included lying to or telling on their friends, hurting them emotionally

*Table 1.1* The six parts story framework

| Main Character: | Environment: | Friends: |
|---|---|---|
| The main character is Buttercup, the rabbit. | She lives in a field full of flowers. It is a windy day and there are clouds in the sky. | Her special friend was Hedgey, the hedgehog. They decided to have a picnic together. |
| *Foes:* | *Challenges:* | *The Outcome:* |
| This is Boa the snake and the problem is that she is jealous of Buttercup and Hedgey's friendship. | Boa wants friends but she is going the wrong way about it.<br><br>What is the right way? | We need to find the right way. |

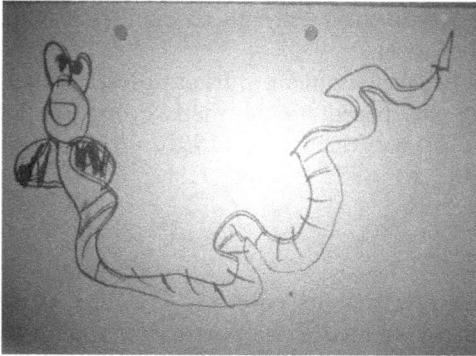

*Figure 1.1* Boa thinking of how to 'get in' to make a lasting friendship

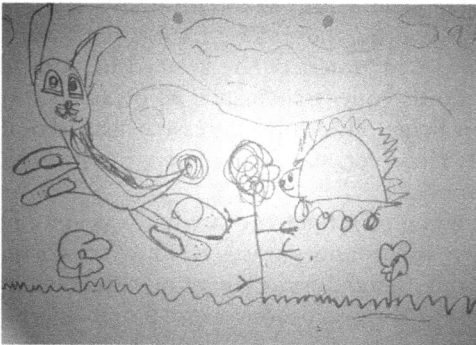

*Figure 1.2* Challenges to maintain friendship

or physically or bullying them. We discussed how hard friendships are to maintain. We talked about what strategies are required to do this.

Three different clay model characters (Buttercup the rabbit, Boa and Hedgey the hedgehog) from the six parts story placed on a multicoloured plate.

Millie expressed a desire to make clay models of the characters in her six-part story (Figure 1.3). She then asked if she could make a short film of her story on her iPad using stop motion to animate the clay models. It was a pleasure to watch her skilfully manipulate each model into separate movements and take the photos with her iPad to create a short stop-go animation. The result was an enchanting film of the three characters dancing and playing joyfully around each other. Millie seemed to be expressing that all she really wanted from friendship was simplicity and togetherness.

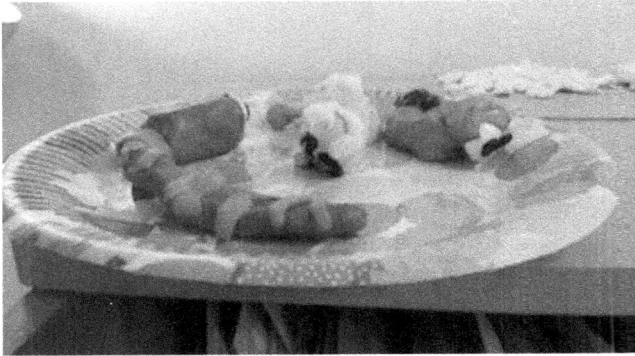

*Figure 1.3* Clay models of the characters in Millie's six-part story

### The Second Phase of Work – Friendships Evolving

Following the filmmaking, I asked her what she would like to work with next and in an enthusiastic rush we began our foray into the Pokémon world (Tajiri, 1996) with an in-depth explanation from Millie. When she started out on her Pokémon journey of discovery, I knew little about this game and found it to be an intensely overwhelming world.

The premise in the mythical world of Pokémon is that young 'trainers' (players) must capture and train over 150 wild creatures in terrains such as Fire, Water, Grass, Thunder and Psychic (Buckingham and Sefton Green 2004). Millie seemed to navigate this world with ease, and it was one where she had an extraordinary knowledge and depth of understanding of. At times it was difficult to keep up with her, a similar experience shared by Davidson (2016). However, I felt we became 'stuck' with the logistics of the game and needed to locate a starting point. I put the suggestion of creating Pokémon lands to Millie and she became enamoured with the idea. She proposed that we lay out three different lands of Thunder, Fire and Water. Millie wanted to dance around the lands once they had been created so for ten minutes we indulged in joyous free dancing. Millie appeared so lively and rejuvenated after this and it seemed to release her to reflect on the next stage of the friendship process. We decided to slow things down in the sessions so that we could absorb all the elements required in obtaining friendship skills. During this process, we began to talk about how we as humans evolve though friendship.

Evaluation was needed to find out not only what we get out of friendships but also what is entailed to make them work. There are a myriad of characters in Pokémon, and this appeared to cloud Millie's process; she became so absorbed in choosing which characters, she might work with but eventually managed to narrow it down to two – Hapne and Evee. Identifying how the characters evolve through friendship Millie explained that it involves petting them, feeding them 'poke puffs', giving them 'Pokémon' beans (which are heart shaped) and stroking them with an 'angelic' feather.

### Third Stage of Work – Feeding the Friendships

At the start of this stage Millie suggested that we create eggs. In our efforts to look after them correctly, we needed to make a nest for them and then cradle and nurture them. We wrote poetic words to the eggs.

Hapne - This egg seems oddly warm. It must be close to hatching.

Eevee - This egg seems so hopeful and full of life. It is ready to burst. So excited.

In the next session, the eggs were warm and about to crack. There was a peaceful and reflective atmosphere in the room as Millie carefully laid out the eggs and Pokémons. She lit a candle and then looking at me steadily began to tear her egg. She said that the hatching of the eggs can happen slowly and then sometimes suddenly it will burst. She then sorted out the conditions they needed to crack which were to create 'steam', to have a nest, play music and dance – and we put these in place. It was really entrancing to witness.

It all felt so calm and nurturing as the egg slowly 'cracked' and Hapne emerged (Figure 1.4). Then Millie helped to burst Eevee's egg laying it gently in the doll's house that was in the room to care for it. She fed it 'citrus berries' and stroked it and played 'peekaboo' with it. She declared 'she likes me' and was rewarded with a stone (which is how you know that a Pokémon likes you). I asked how it felt in her body and she said, 'so warm and good'.

The next task was to look after the hatchlings and Millie organised a tea party for them where they ate 'poke puffs' and she played ball and hide and seek with them.

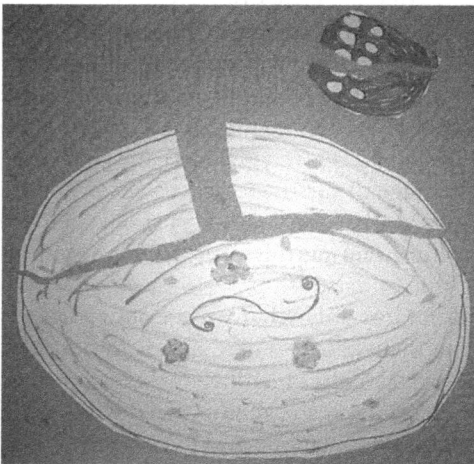

Figure 1.4 The hatchlings

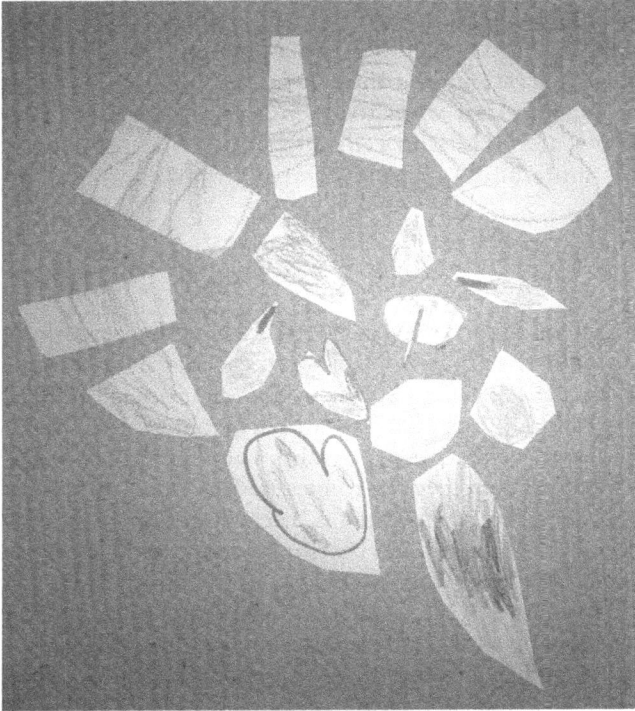

*Figure 1.5* Recipe for a special food for the hatchlings

She then decided to create a special food for them and came up with this recipe (Figure 1.5):

Berries

Poke beans

Special poke bean treats

Stinky but tasty essence from vile plume flowers

Water type's water

1/2 an eggshell from a big egg

Grass from the cloak and grass types

Together we 'mixed up' the food from the recipe and then set up two bowls and spoons for us to feed Eevee and Hapne. She sang to the hatchlings as she fed them and then made beds for them to sleep in. During this feeding ritual, it was as though Millie was absorbing the appreciation of the fact that it was not just about having things done to her in friendship; it was also about the actions that she could do for others. She enjoyed embodying the satisfying feelings that follow when we accomplish these things.

I detected the beginnings of an understanding of reciprocation in friendship. At the end of the session, just as we were leaving to go back to class, Millie turned to me and enquired, 'Do you remember when I was in a little group – I liked that' (She had been in a small social skills group during Year 2). I asked if she would like to be in group again and she answered enthusiastically, 'Yes!' adding thoughtfully, 'sometimes I want to be on my own and sometimes I want to be in a group'. Millie's sentiments echo findings by Calder Hill and Pellicano (2013) that the autistic notion of friendship is more about sharing company than sharing emotions.

## Discussion

Originating from an idea mooted by Conn (2014), I have been working for several years with inclusive groups of neurotypical and neurodiverse boys and girls (Pomeroy, 2016; Dyer, 2017) to aid their social skills. I have found these to be mutually beneficial to all participants. I devised a theory that to achieve a more effective approach to understanding social ability for the autistic person, there needed to be a period when they work individually in the therapeutic space. Using a variety of dramatherapy techniques – as outlined in Millie's intervention – they could explore, experiment, discard and integrate the knowledge and requirements for securing friends (Gus, 2000; Conn, 2016). The most rewarding thing about this intervention was the different aspects of dramatherapy – drawing, filmmaking, dancing, storytelling, ritual and drama work etc. – that were utilised in achieving the desired outcome for Millie, as well as the provision of flexibility and modification in the structure to engage her.

The pace of the intervention and activities in the sessions would be led by the young person and they would have agency and choice throughout this process, a principle also advocated by other dramatherapists (e.g., Ramsden, 2017). The anticipated outcome would be that the young person would then voice their desire to be in a group independently, when they felt ready to do so. Endeavouring to provide therapy in schools where there are many demands on time – with the added factor of terms and school holidays – can be vexing. Taking this into consideration, I felt that I skilfully used the school year to the best advantage to result in the desired outcome (De Geest and Meganck, 2019). Millie's needs necessitated the application of a gentle and unhurried pace so that her exploration of the two-way process in friendship would be firmly secured. The acquisition of strategies to counter any difficulties that might arise within a friendship with a calm mind-set was also pivotal for Millie.

When undertaking the literature review for this case study, one goal comes sharply into focus – there seems to be a requirement for girl-only support groups where the autistic female is offered space for activities that have communication and emotional connection as the main feature

(Carpenter et al., 2019). Receiving mentoring from older autistic women who have been through similar experiences could be factored in (Cook and Garnett, 2018). Interestingly, Rosqvist, Brownlow and O'Dell (2015) note that the specific aim of social groups should be to encourage friendships and close relationships in an environment that is relaxing and enjoyable, rather than the autistic person managing neurotypical world ideals. As Dix (2016) noted, dramatherapy groups can offer a safe space to foster such genuine connections and empower the voices of autistic girls.

## Conclusion

Millie's embodied understanding and a growing realisation that she was 'looking after the hatchlings' was the most crucial and poignant aspect of this intervention. Her genuine pleasure, and the satisfaction she felt at the revelation that she was able to give to others rather than be given to, was a delight to witness. The flexible, embodied and playful nature of the dramatherapy was very apparent in the work with Millie. Moving into a managed group supported her to try out what she had embodied in 1:1 dramatherapy in a nurturing group environment with empathetic peers before taking it out into the social world. Her developing confidence enabled her to ask, of her own volition, to be in a group – something I was not expecting to happen - and this gave me the validation that my theory had worked. However, it is only about one autistic girl. In trying to explore the efficacy of my theory, I have applied it to other interventions with young people on the autistic spectrum with successful results. This growing practice-based evidence warrants the suggestion that future research is needed to explore the impact and implications of dramatherapy in a wider context.

## Acknowledgements

I want to thank Millie and her family for granting me the enormous privilege of working in close partnership with them.

This chapter is written in memory of Millie's mother who died six months after the intervention ended. She always encouraged me enthusiastically to write about autism.

I would also like to extend my gratitude to the entirely unique and innovative primary school where this intervention took place.

## References

American Psychiatric Association (2013) *Diagnostic and statistical manual of mental disorders*. Washington, DC: Am. Psychiatry. Publ. 5th ed.
Attwood, T. (2007) *The complete guide to Asperger's syndrome*. Pbk. Ed edition. London; Philadelphia: Jessica Kingsley Publishers.

Attwood, T. and Garnett. (2022) 'Why camouflage autism? Attwood and Garnett Events'. Available at: https://attwoodandgarnettevents.com/whycamouflageautism?.

Autism Speaks (2021) 'What is the DSM-5 diagnostic criteria for autism?' Available at: https://www.autismspeaks.org/autism-diagnosis-criteria-dsm-5.

Bargiela, D.S. (2019) *Camouflage: The hidden lives of autistic women.* Illustrated edition. London: Jessica Kingsley Publishers.

Bruzzese, F. (Producer), Parry, M. and Olb, J. (Directors) (2018) Nanette Australian Netflix

Bukowski, W.M. Newcomb, A.F. and Hartup, W. (1996) *The company they keep: Friendship in childhood and adolescence* (1996). New York, NY, US: Cambridge University Press (The company they keep: Friendship in childhood and adolescence), pp. x, 426.

Bullivant, F.F. (2018) *Working with girls and young women with an autism spectrum condition: A practical guide for clinicians.* London; Philadelphia: Jessica Kingsley Publishers.

Bauminger, N., Shulman, C. and Agam, G. (2003) 'Peer interaction and loneliness in high-functioning children with autism', *Journal of Autism and Developmental Disorders*, 33(5), pp. 489–507. Available at: 10.1023/A:1025827427901.

Calder, L., Hill, V. and Pellicano, E. (2013) '"Sometimes I want to play by myself": Understanding what friendship means to children with autism in mainstream primary schools', *Autism: The International Journal of Research and Practice*, 17(3), pp. 296–316. Available at: 10.1177/1362361312467866.

Carpenter, B., Happé, F., Egerton, J. and Hollins, B.S. (eds.) (2019)*Educational, family and personal perspectives.* London: Routledge. Available at: 10.4324/9781351234429.

Cook, B. and Garnett, M. (2018) *Spectrum women: Walking to the beat of autism.* Jessica Kingsley Publishers.

Conn, C. (2014) *A sociocultural perspective on theory and practice.* London: Routledge. Available at:10.4324/9781315795454.

Conn, C. (2016) *Play and friendship in inclusive autism education: Supporting learning and development.* 1st edn. London; New York: Routledge.

Daniel, L.S. and Billingsley, B.S. (2010) 'What boys with an autism spectrum disorder say about establishing and maintaining friendships', *Focus on Autism and Other Developmental Disabilities*, 25(4), pp. 220–229. Available at: 10.1177/1088357610378290.

Davidson, R. (2016) 'Entering colourland: Working with metaphor with high functioning autistic children', in D. Haythorne and A. Seymour (eds.) *Dramatherapy and Autism.* Routledge, pp. 16–29.

Dean, M., Harwood, R. and Kasari, C. (2017) 'The art of camouflage: Gender differences in the social behaviors of girls and boys with autism spectrum disorder', *Autism: The International Journal of Research and Practice*, 21(6), pp. 678–689. Available at: 10.1177/1362361316671845.

De Geest, R. and Meganck, R. (2019) 'How do time limits affect our psychotherapies? A literature review', *Psychologica Belgica*, 59(1), p. 1. Available at: 10.5334/pb.475.

Disney, W. (Producer) and Hand, D. (Director) (1942) Bambi (Film) American RKO Radio Pictures.

Dix, A. (2016) 'Becoming visible: Identifying and Empowering girls on the autistic spectrum through dramatherapy', in D. Haythorne and A. Seymour (eds.) *Dramatherapy and autism*. London: Routledge, pp. 66–80.

Dyer, N. (2017) 'Behold the tree: An exploration of the social integration of boys on the autistic spectrum in a mainstream primary school through a dramatherapy intervention', *Dramatherapy*, 38(2–3), pp. 80–93. Available at: 10.1080/0263 0672.2017.1329845.

Eaton, J. (2017) *A guide to mental health issues in girls and young women on the autism spectrum: Diagnosis, intervention and family support*. Jessica Kingsley Publishers.

Gadsby, H. (2022) Ten Steps to Nanette - a Memoir Situation Allen & Unwin

Gould, J and Ashton-Smith, J. (2011) 'Missed diagnosis or misdiagnosis? Girls and women on the autism spectrum', *Good Autism Practice (GAP)*, 12(1), pp. 34–41.

Gus, L. (2000) 'Autism: Promoting peer understanding', *Educational Psychology in Practice*, 16(4), pp. 461–468.

Happé, F. and Frith, U. (1995) Theory of mind in autism, *Learning and cognition in autism*, pp. 177–197.

Hiller, R.M., Young, R.L., and Weber, N. (2014) 'Sex differences in autism spectrum disorder based on DSM-5 criteria: Evidence from clinician and teacher reporting', *Journal of Abnormal Child Psychology*, 42, pp. 1381–1393. Available at: 10.1007/s10802-014-9881-x.

Hendrickx, S. (2015) *Women and girls with autism spectrum disorder: Understanding life experiences from early childhood to old age*. Jessica Kingsley Publishers.

Hughes, A.M. (2017) *Making friends: How the friendly group supports children and young people on the autism spectrum*. Worth Publishing Limited.

Hull, L., Petrides, K.V., Allison, C., Smith, P., Baron-Cohen, S., Lai, M.-C. and Mandy, W. (2017) '"Putting on my best normal": Social camouflaging in adults with autism spectrum conditions', *Journal of Autism and Developmental Disorders*, 47(8), pp. 2519–2534. Available at: 10.1007/s10803-017-3166-5.

Lahad, M. (1992) 'Six-piece story-making and BASIC Ph', in *Dramatherapy: Theory and practice 2*. 2nd edn. London and New York: Routledge.

May, K. (2019) *The electricity of every living thing: A woman's walk in the wild to find her way home*. Trapeze.

Meldrum, B. (1994) 'Evaluation and assessment in dramatherapy', in S. Jennings, A. Cattanach, S. Mitchell, A. Chesner and B. Meldrum (eds.) *The Handbook of Dramatherapy*. London: Routledge, pp. 185–206.

Milner, V., McIntosh, H., Colvert, E. and Happé, F (2019) 'A qualitative exploration of the female experience of autism spectrum disorder (ASD)', *Journal of Autism and Developmental Disorders*, 49(6), pp. 2389–2402. Available at: 10.1007/s10803-019-03906-4.

Moyse, R. and Porter, J. (2015) 'The experience of the hidden curriculum for autistic girls at mainstream primary schools', *European Journal of Special Needs Education*, 30(2), pp. 187–201. Available at: 10.1080/08856257.2014.986915.

Nessen, C. (Producers) Grossman, N. (Director) (2020 September 10th) I am Greta British BBC A Hula Original Documentary

NICE (2011) *Overview | Autism spectrum disorder in under 19s: recognition, referral and diagnosis | Guidance |*. NICE. Available at: https://www.nice.org.uk/guidance/cg128 (Accessed: 28 January 2023).

Pomeroy, R.A. (2016) *Improv for autism: Using theatre to teach social communication skills to children and youth with autism.* Maseter's Dissertation. California State University.

Ramsden, E. (2017) 'Supporting agency, choice making and the expression of 'voice' with Kate: Dramatherapy in a mainstream school with a 9-year-old girl diagnosed with ASD and ADHD', in D. Haythorne and A. Seymour (eds.) *Dramatherapy and Autism.* Routledge, pp. 53–65.

Rosqvist, H.B., Brownlow, C. and O'Dell, L. (2015) '"What's the point of having friends?": Reformulating Notions of the meaning of friends and friendship among autistic people', *Disability Studies Quarterly*, 35(4). Available at: 10.18061/dsq.v35i4.3254.

Roth, I., Barson, C., Hoekstra, R., Pasco, G. and Whatson, T. (2010) *The autism spectrum in the 21st century: Exploring psychology, biology and practice.* London/Philadelphia: Jessica Kingsley Publishers. Available at: http://www.jkp.com/catalogue/book/9781849050876 (Accessed 28 January 2023).

Rourke, A. (2019) 'Greta Thunberg responds to Asperger's critics: 'It's a superpower' The Guardian News & Media Group'. Available at: https://www.theguardian.com/environment/2019/sep/02/greta-thunberg-responds-to-aspergers-critics-its-a-superpower (Retrieved January 2021).

Tajiri, S. (1996) *Pokémon, Nintendo.* Tokyo, Japan.

Tierney, S., Burns, J. and Kilbey, E. (2016) 'Looking behind the mask: Social coping strategies of girls on the autistic spectrum', *Research in Autism Spectrum Disorders*, 23, pp. 73–83. Available at: 10.1016/j.rasd.2015.11.013.

Whitlock, A., Fulton, K., Lai, M.-C., Pellicano, E. and Mandy, W. (2020) 'Recognition of girls on the autism spectrum by primary school educators: An experimental study', *Autism Research*, 13(8), pp. 1358–1372. Available at: 10.1002/aur.2316.

# Chapter 2

# Fostering Creative Social Connections Between Autistic Children and Their Families Through Shared Music Experiences

*Grace Thompson*

## Introduction

Music therapists began to document their work with autistic children[1] in the 1950s (Reschke-Hernandez, 2011), with various practitioners observing that autistic children showed an interest in music and movement. In those early days of the music therapy profession, practitioners proposed that they could offer a distinct opportunity for people with diverse forms of communication to feel connected and understood, without relying on words. Even though many music therapists worked in institutional settings at this time (Nordoff and Robbins, 1977), early innovators such as Juliette Alvin described how music therapists could also consult with families and include them in the child's sessions (Alvin, 1978). Autism is hallmarked by differences in social interaction behaviours and preferences, and often the individual also has unique sensory sensitivities and experiences (American Psychiatric Association, 2013; Walker, 2014). While these differences can be challenging for non-autistic family members to interpret and understand, music therapy research has found that shared music experiences can foster stronger relationships and interactive play between diverse family members (Allgood, 2005; Thompson et al., 2014).

Before discussing how music therapy can support autistic children and their families, I will begin by positioning my own practice and research. I have been a registered music therapist since 1994 and strive to follow the child's interests and facilitate music experiences that feel like a natural part of their play routines. I am also a person with a significant physical disability that required approximately 12 major surgeries in my childhood before the age of 13. I have lived experience of being separated from my parents while in hospital as a young child, feeling isolated and unable to express the complex emotions I was feeling.

DOI: 10.4324/9781003201656-4

My own disabled identity helps me to listen deeply to the experiences of autistic people and I strive to honour a key tenant of the disability rights movement: nothing about us without us (Charlton, 1998). It is therefore important to sincerely acknowledge that more and more autistic people are sharing their stories about the therapy they received as children, with some describing distressing and confronting memories of oppression and abuse (Bascom, 2012). Throughout this chapter, I will attempt to use language that is respectful and balanced. I endeavour to align with autistic authors who compel researchers to avoid focussing on ableist therapy outcomes, such as promoting 'appropriate' eye contact, and instead design participatory projects that support autistic children's autonomy and agency (Bottema-Beutel et al., 2021). For example, much has been written about the deficits of autistic children's play (Baron-Cohen, 1987); however, these understandings are often viewed from a neurotypical perspective. Autistic advocates have instead highlighted the strengths in autistic children's preferred play styles, such as their focussed attention to detail (Ludwig, 2020). These social justice considerations need to be part of our practice and research because, despite the advances made in education and inclusion, autistic people continue to report experiencing discrimination and social isolation (Jones et al., 2018). Therefore, we must confront the growing realisation that attitudes of non-autistic people are likely to be a significant barrier to social inclusion (den Houting, 2019).

### Theoretical Foundations for Music Therapy with Autistic Children and Their Families

When working with families, partnership models such as family-centred practice (Dunst and Trivette, 2009) acknowledge that the people we work with are the experts in their own lives. Early childhood practitioners have therefore advocated for collaborative approaches that strive to enable and empower families and parents. This trend is also reflected in literature describing music therapy practice approaches. An international survey of 125 music therapists working with families revealed that 93.6% include family members as active participants in sessions with their child, and a small percentage (4.8%) described providing separate sessions for adult family members (Tuomi et al., 2021).

While music therapists work with families who have children of various ages, the first eight years of a child's life are often a time when family involvement is at a peak. In the early years, children rely on their family to scaffold their daily routines, relationships and play. The relational security provided by parents[2] is therefore vital to their overall development (Stern, 1985). The early years are also a time when all children use a variety of communication strategies in their play and interactions. While language and symbolic communication are emerging, children and parents must also include other forms of expression in their day-to-day interactions.

Two theories from scholars with backgrounds encompassing music, psychology and psychoanalysis describe these other forms of expression in musical terms: communicative musicality (Trevarthen and Malloch, 2000); and forms of vitality (Stern, 2010). Both theories also highlight the developmental importance of emotionally attuned, playful and plentiful interactions between children and their parents.

Daniel Stern's theory, forms of vitality, grew from his earlier research into responsive and emotionally attuned parent-infant interactions (Stern, 1985). Stern observed that parents tried to attune to their child through cross modal forms such as vocal intonation and rhythmic movements that did not require the child to understand the words they spoke. Through these musical elements, the parent can communicate their interpretation of the infant's emotions or actions, invite them into longer interactive play experiences, or provide comfort and security. The infant is then believed to experience that their emotions and actions can be shared with others, and so their social communication development expands (Stern, 2010). Communicative musicality is a theory that also emerged from analysing video footage of parent-infant interaction (Trevarthen and Malloch, 2000). The microanalysis revealed that parents and infants primarily engaged with each other using musical elements of pitch (changes in the melodic contour of the voice), timbre (changes in the quality of the voice), pulse (changes in rhythm) and narrative (the overall form of the interaction).

Forms of vitality and communicative musicality are theories based on general development, rather than being autism specific. However, given that parent-child interactions are the primary means of scaffolding relational learning, the capacity of the parent to attune and respond to their autistic child is expected to have similar developmental implications (Ammaniti and Ferrari, 2013). Music therapists working with families often base their work on the understanding that fostering the quality of parent-child responsiveness through enjoyable and playful musical interactions may provide an important foundation to maximise child development and strengthen family relationships (Tuomi et al., 2021). Music therapy theorist Carolyn Kenny (1989) highlighted the importance of music-based play to support creativity, identity formation and relationship. Kenny's (1989) theory, the field of play, proposes that a musical play space shared with an attuned therapist can create a supportive environment for change and growth. A growing body of research provides support for this theoretical stance by investigating how music-based experiences influence the quality of play between parents and their autistic children (Hernandez-Ruiz, 2020; Lense et al., 2020; Thompson et al., 2019).

## Study Approach

Qualitative research methods have helped to build the evidence base of family-centred music therapy practice by providing insight into the parent experience and advancing our understanding of the benefits and challenges of this approach. My own research has adopted a theoretical basis informed by Moustakas's and Giorgi's notion of examining the person centred experience of a phenomenon, often referred to as descriptive phenomenology (Moustakas, 1994). Descriptive phenomenology typically begins with an in-depth interview that invites the participant to openly describe their experiences of a phenomenon. The researcher then seeks to dwell upon the data to explore possible meanings and themes, and finally constructs a rich description that captures the essence of the phenomenon (Finlay, 2014).

In this chapter, I am revisiting the findings from two of my previous qualitative inquiries to propose a framework for how music therapists can support parents to support their children by working within family-centred principles. The first study included 11 mothers whose children were diagnosed with autism. The children ranged in age between three and six years, and included eight boys and three girls. The children spoke limited words at the start of the study and were attending a family-centred early childhood intervention programme. Three of the 11 mothers spoke English as a second language, and one was a single parent. Five of the mothers' highest level of education was 11–12 years, five mothers had completed professional training courses and one mother had a university degree. Three of the eleven mothers considered themselves to be under financial stress. Each family participated in 16 weekly family-centred music therapy sessions, where parents were supported to join in the music-based play. The music therapy methods aimed to create opportunities for reciprocal personal interactions, affect sharing, turn-taking and joint attention (Thompson and McFerran, 2015).

The second study was a follow up with this same cohort four years later. The parents were invited to have a further interview to explore their perspectives on the long-term value of participating in the family-centred sessions (Thompson, 2017). Eight mothers participated, with family demographics being very similar to the first study. Both studies were approved by the University of Melbourne Human Research Ethics Committee.

## Findings

The qualitative analysis across these two studies highlighted that these mothers perceived a combination of benefits for their children and for themselves. In the first study, which immediately followed their participation in the 16-week music therapy programme, all mothers described changes in the way they responded to and related to their children. Some described how simply increasing the quantity of play-based interactions in their daily routine helped them to feel more connected to their children. Other mothers felt closer to their child during the music-based play because there was a shared sense of enjoyment in these interactions. Lastly, others described a profound experience of deep connection with their child through music-based play that they considered strengthened their bond. The analysis revealed that these changes in the experience of closeness in their relationship had flow-on consequences for the way they perceived and responded to their child (Thompson and McFerran, 2015).

In the follow up study four years later, mothers described that these changes in their relationship, perception, and responses to their child had continued well beyond the period of the initial study. These findings suggest that the benefits of an intensive period of family-centred music therapy can continue through to the child's first years of school. In reflecting on their experiences, many mothers described how seeing a different side to their child within music-based play helped them to engage their child more successfully in many other activities. Monica described her experience as follows:

> My daughter was very active back then. I don't know how to say it ... she was just not settled at all. She was all over the place. When we found out she liked the music instruments, we would put the instruments everywhere on the floor and she would just play with them for maybe 30 minutes or more. She never had interest in other toys, books. Never, nothing. In the early days when you find something your child is interested in, it's like, oh my gosh. Now, I know her interests, I signed her up for dancing classes next. I really can see joy when I see her in the dancing classes and when she is singing, so now I know that's ... that's her thing.

Another key theme in this follow-up study revealed that participating together in music provides a rare opportunity for mutual enjoyment between mother and child. These mutually enjoyable interactions did not just occur during the original music therapy sessions, but they continued for all the mothers interviewed in the follow up. Maria described,

> Even after 4 years, my daughter still brings out the instruments. She gives the drum to me, the cymbals to her dad, the little shaker things to her sister. She tells us when to start and when to stop. So we all play at the same time (laughs). We make a lot of noise really, but she's always initiating the play, so ... that's huge.

When the interviewer asked Maria how this makes her feel, she said:

> Really good, because she's coming to us. She's seeking us. My daughter would normally only come to me to ask for something. But, with the music therapy, it was enjoying time with me, with mum. It wasn't about 'make me a sandwich' or, 'I want this or that'. And it made me feel good because we had a mother-child connection, so that was really nice for me.

When reflecting on the benefits for their children, some mothers described the importance of providing opportunities for the child to express their emotions and personality through music. For those children who were non-speaking or whose forms of communication were difficult for others to interpret, some mothers particularly highlighted that these opportunities were uncommon. Sarah described her growing understanding of the importance of self-expression as follows:

> I can see the joy in my son's face when he's getting to express himself. He spends a lot of his life not being able to express himself, and not being acknowledged for the intelligence he has. The music kind of fostered that individual sense of self, and that is something that doesn't get talked about enough in disability in general and it needs to. I think it's only now that I can step back and really see the importance of fostering his interests and supporting his self-expression.

## Discussion

When looking across descriptions of music therapists' approach to working with families in the literature, three characteristics have been identified: (1) prioritising the quality of interactions between family members; (2) being respectful of the family's knowledge, wishes and resources; and (3) promoting the sustainable use of music that can continue without input from the music therapist (Jacobsen and Thompson, 2016). However, these characteristics all focus on the family system and the therapeutic alliance. There are other considerations for working with families, such as broader societal values, that are likely to influence the reasons families seek therapy for their child in the first place, and the way goals are identified.

### Reflections on Family-Centred Music Therapy

Family-centred practitioners, as described earlier, strive to enable and empower families and parents. This ethos suggests that there are broader factors that contribute to the success of therapy that go beyond the discipline-specific methods that the therapist applies. Looking back over these findings, I have continued to reflect on my overarching therapeutic aim, which is to support the parent to support the child. The family's needs and resources are likely to change over time, and so the therapist must consider how to approach their work to provide the preferred level of support for the family. The way therapists provide this support is nuanced and multifaceted, which I have come to understand as a continuum that is fluid and responsive. I have attempted to represent how the therapeutic alliance between the therapist and parent might evolve or change over time in Figure 2.1.

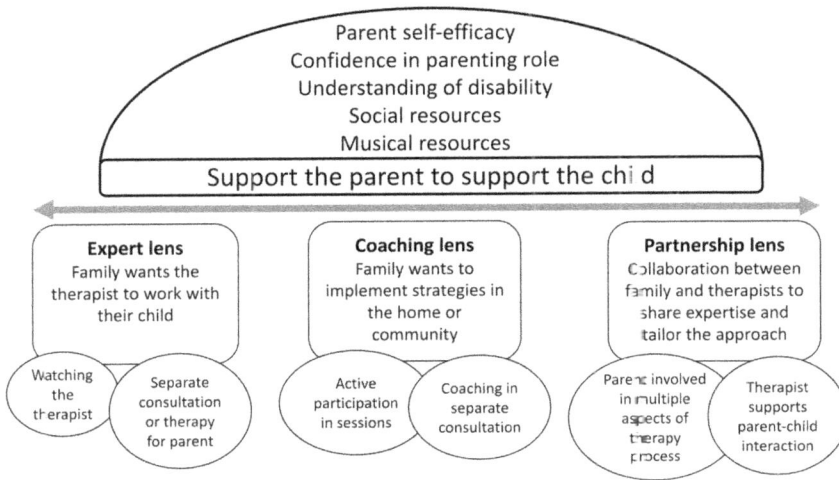

*Figure 2.1* A continuum of support when working with families

Many therapists who work with families emphasise the importance of respect and understanding for the family's context (Jacobsen and Thompson, 2016). Represented by the arch at the top of Figure 2.1, various facets should be considered, such as the parents' sense of self-efficacy, their confidence in the parenting role, their understanding of their child's condition, their understanding of disability more generally and their social and musical resources.

Following on, the facilitation approach, or lens, that the therapist takes should be sensitive to the fact that not all families wish to actively participate in their child's music therapy sessions at all times. For example, parents might choose to have their own music-oriented counselling sessions where they can focus on their emotional needs and consult with the music therapist about how to support their child at home (Gottfried, 2016). Following these separate counselling sessions, parents have reported feeling empowered; they also have observed flow-on benefits for their child's wellbeing and family quality of life (Blauth, 2019). From the perspective of the continuum of support, it seems that these separate consultation and counselling sessions can merge into coaching. For example, parents receiving separate sessions with the music therapist might also review video footage of their child's therapy sessions and discuss ways to incorporate strategies into everyday life (Blauth, 2019; Gottfried, 2016).

While both active parent involvement in music therapy sessions and separate parent counselling can build the capacity of parents to incorporate strategies at home without the therapist being present, there are distinct parent coaching models now emerging in music therapy. Parent coaching or parent-mediated approaches begin from the premise of building the capacity of parents to use specific therapy techniques and strategies independently with their child (Hernandez-Ruiz, 2020). While the focus of coaching models is often on improving the child's developmental outcomes, benefits for parents are also documented such as improved self-efficacy and parent-responsiveness (Teggelove et al., 2019).

Working in partnership with families is multifaceted. At times, the music therapist might directly model techniques and strategies which could be seen as aligned with an expert model. Within the session, the therapist might also share their knowledge of theories and child development principles, and support the parent to lead music experiences within the session similar to a coaching approach. At other times, the parent and therapist might actively share expertise and collaboratively design music-based experiences to meet family-identified goals. Therefore, partnership approaches are typically more fluid and dynamic as the therapist strives to build the capacity of the parent to support their child using music. Qualitative research has shown that following involvement in family-centred music therapy, parents placed greater value on play with their autistic child and better understood their child's strengths and interests. Parents also describe feeling more confident when interacting with their child, and more pleasure in the mutual play interactions (Allgood, 2005; Thompson, 2017; Thompson and McFerran, 2015).

### Therapy in the Context of Autistic Advocacy

Several music therapy researchers and practitioners have sought to reflect on their role within the context of disability studies. For example, Susan Hadley (2014) questioned her own desire to 'help' disabled people without challenging societal notions of pathology and the flow-on ruling norms that position disabled people as 'problematic'. Ethnomusicologist and musician Michael Bakan challenges music therapists' world view of disability, stating that even when music therapists highlight 'autistic strengths and [place] emphasis on success-directed orientations, the goal of the enterprise remains essentially unaffected: solve problems, reduce symptoms, increase functionality' (Bakan, 2014, para. 4). Hadley and Bakan's commentaries raise ethical questions around the process of identifying goals for autistic children, such as who decides on the goal and what the focus of the goal should be.

In my own research with families who have newly diagnosed children, I have observed that the family's understanding of disability can impact the way they engage with therapy services. Some might be very focused on functional skills such as speaking clearly or turn taking, others might want their child to find something they enjoy and are good at, and others may seek a combination of goals. Autistic advocates call for society to accept autistic ways of being rather than solely focusing on changing the autistic individual

(Bascom, 2012; Walker, 2014). Ne'eman (2021) proposes that, rather than seeking to reduce diagnostic traits that are 'stigmatized by not harmful' (p. 569), therapists should instead focus on prioritising the 'underlying goal of communication' (p. 570) where various modes for communication are valued.

The discourse led by autistic advocates and, increasingly, autistic music therapists, requires a deep level of reflexivity into our practice ethics. The qualitative data from the studies described in this chapter revealed other possibilities for music therapy, such as fostering family quality of life (Thompson and McFerran, 2015), which is somewhat better aligned with calls from advocates to accept autistic people's ways of being (Leza, 2020). It is therefore important to note that many of the outcomes parents described following music therapy include creating an environment where all family members can participate, and parents gaining new insight into their child's strengths, abilities and interests. Parents further described how having a better understanding of their child has also improved the quality of their relationship. The nuanced ways that parent and child wellbeing intertwine is reflected in research findings that show how a parent's mental health impacts the way they view and interpret their child's behaviour (Bennett et al., 2012).

Navigating our own beliefs and values as therapists alongside supporting families to support their children, and at the same time facilitating music experiences that are meaningful for the child, is at the heart of the family-centred practitioner's skill. However, perhaps these complexities are also at the heart of systems theory itself: understanding the impact of the macro-system (the values and attitudes of culture and society) on the microsystems of the family or school, and the ways that microsystems interact together (the mesosystem) (Bronfenbrenner, 1979). Leaning into the theories that inform my practice, I have therefore fashioned a meta-aim for my work: to nurture the development of attuned and secure family relationships in order to maximise the autistic child's opportunity for meaningful connections with others.

Lastly, while deeply reflective perspectives from parents have led to important practice developments, an important perspective is missing in the research to date: that of the children themselves. While collecting qualitative data from young children is challenging and requires a great deal of plan-ning and consideration, participatory research that does not include the voices of key stakeholders is ultimately limited. One example from music therapy that comes close to including the perspectives of child participants is the documentary film titled 'Operation Syncopation' (M. Thompson, 2017). This film tells the story of ten families who received music therapy from Amelia Oldfield 16 years prior. The film's director, Maxim Thompson, was himself one of the child-participants. With original film footage from the children's sessions interwoven with reflections from the parents and their now adult children, this documentary could be viewed as arts-based research. At the end of the film, Maxim poignantly reflects that attending music therapy as a child was just his 'job', and he perceived that the real benefit of the music therapy sessions was for his parents. The director's retrospective views are important, challenging, and point to the need for more representation of children's perspectives in future research concerned with family outcomes. Participatory research which includes autistic children's perspectives may go some way towards co-creating therapy services that are respectful of the child's unique autistic ways of being.

## Notes

1   I choose to use identity-first language throughout this chapter to acknowledge the preference of many autistic people who use this terminology to reduce stigma and foster pride.
2   I use the term 'parent' throughout this chapter to refer to the child's primary caregiver, not just their biological parent.

## References

Allgood, N. (2005) 'Parents' perceptions of family-based group music therapy for children with autism spectrum disorders', *Music Therapy Perspectives*, 23, pp. 92–99.

Alvin, J. (1978) *Music therapy for the autistic child*. Oxford University Press.

American Psychiatric Association. (2013) *Diagnostic and statistical manual of mental disorders –DSM-5* (5th edn.). American Psychiatric Publishing.

Ammaniti, M. and Ferrari, P. (2013) 'Vitality affects in Daniel Stern's thinking – A psychological and neurobiological perspective', *Infant Mental Health Journal*, 34(5), pp. 367–375. Available at: https://www.ncbi.nlm.nih.gov/pmc/articles/PMC4278751/

Bakan, M.B. (2014) 'Ethnomusicological perspectives on autism, neurodiversity, and music therapy', *Voices: A World Forum for Music Therapy*, 14(3). Retrieved 4 September 2016, from https://voices.no/index.php/voices/article/view/799

Baron-Cohen, S. (1987) 'Autism and symbolic play', *British Journal of Developmental Psychology*, 5(2), pp. 139–148.

Bascom, J. (2012) *Loud hands: Autistic people, speaking*. Autistic Press.

Bennett, T., Boyle, M., Georgiades, K., Georgiades, S., Thompson, A., Duku, E., Bryson, S., Fombonne, E., Vaillancourt, T. and Zwaigenbaum, L. (2012) 'Influence of reporting effects on the association between maternal depression and child autism spectrum disorder behaviors', *Journal of Child Psychology and Psychiatry*, 53(1), pp. 89–96. 10.1111/j.1469-7610.2011.02451.x

Blauth, L. (2019) *Music therapy and parent counselling to enhance resilience in young children with autism spectrum disorder: A mixed methods study*. Anglia Ruskin University. https://arro.anglia.ac.uk/id/eprint/704640/

Bottema-Beutel, K., Kapp, S.K., Lester, J.N., Sasson, N.J. and Hand, B.N. (2021) 'Avoiding ableist language: Suggestions for autism researchers', *Autism in Adulthood*, 3(1), pp. 18–29. 10.1089/aut.2020.0014

Bronfenbrenner, U. (1979) *The ecology of human development: Experiments by nature and design*. Harvard University Press.

Charlton, J.I. (1998) *Nothing about us without us*. University of California Press.

den Houting, J. (2019) 'Neurodiversity: An insider's perspective', *Autism*, 23(2), pp. 271–273. 10.1177/1362361318820

Dunst, C.J. and Trivette, C. (2009) 'Capacity-building family-systems intervention practices', *Journal of Family Social Work*, 12(2), pp. 119–143. 10.1080/10522150802713322

Finlay, L. (2014) 'Engaging phenomenological analysis', *Qualitative Research in Psychology*, 11(2), pp. 121–141. 10.1080/14780887.2013.807899

Gottfried, T. (2016) 'Music-oriented counselling model for parents of children with autism spectrum disorder', in S. Lindahl Jacobsen and G. Thompson (Eds.) *Music therapy with families: Therapeutic approaches and theoretical perspectives*. Jessica Kingsley Publishers, pp. 116–134.

Hadley, S.J. (2014) 'Shifting frames: Are we really embracing human diversities?', *Voices: A World Forum for Music Therapy*, 14(3).

Hernandez-Ruiz, E. (2020) 'Parent coaching of music interventions for children with ASD: A conceptual framework', *Nordic Journal of Music Therapy*, 29(3), pp. 200–221. 10.1080/08098131.2019.1647447

Jacobsen, S.L. and Thompson, G. (2016) 'Working with families: Emerging characteristics', in S.L. Jacobson and G. Thompson (Eds.) *Music therapy with families. Therapeutic approaches & theoretical perspectives*. Jessica Kingsley.

Jones, S., Akram, M., Murphy, N., Myers, P. and Vickers, N. (2018) *Community attitudes & behaviours towards autism; and experiences of autistic people and their families: General awareness, knowledge and understanding of autism and social isolation*. AMAZE website http://www.onethingforautism.com.au/wp-content/uploads/2018/05/Autism-research-report-General-awareness-knowledge-and-understanding-of-autism-and-social-isolation-1.pdf

Kenny, C.B. (1989) *The field of play: A guide for the theory and practice of music therapy*. Ridgeview.

Lense, M.D., Beck, S., Liu, C., Pfeiffer, R., Diaz, N., Lynch, M., Goodman, N., Summers, A. and Fisher, M.H. (2020) 'Parents, peers, and musical play: Integrated parent-child music class program supports community participation and well-being for families of children with and without autism spectrum disorder', *Frontiers in Psychology*, 11, p. 2775.

Leza, J. (2020) 'Neuroqueering music therapy: Observations on the current state of neurodiversity in music therapy practice', in D. Milton (ed.) *The neurodiversity reader*. Pavilion, pp. 210–225.

Ludwig, F.L. (2020) *Pathologising autism*. http://franklludwig.com/pathologisingautism.html?fbclid=IwAR2jROjqIUuj3YDR%20UygepISyjv8uz%20hJblh4G9hwdYF-sZ9c98Fx8YAxYeZA

Moustakas, C. (1994) *Phenomenological research methods*. SAGE Publications.

Ne'eman, A. (2021) 'When disability Is defined by behavior, outcome measures should not promote "passing"', *AMA Journal of Ethics*, 23(7), pp. 569–575. 10.1001/amajethics.2021.569

Nordoff, P. and Robbins, C. (1977). *Creative music therapy: Individualized treatment for the handicapped child*. John Day Co.

Reschke-Hernandez, A. (2011) 'History of music therapy treatment interventions for children with autism', *Journal of Music Therapy*, 48(2), pp. 169–207. 10.1093/jmt/48.2.169

Stern, D.N. (1985) *The interpersonal world of the infant*. Basic Books Inc.

Stern, D.N. (2010) *Forms of vitality*. Oxford University Press.

Teggelove, K., Thompson, G. and Tamplin, J. (2019) 'Supporting positive parenting practices within a community-based music therapy group program: Pilot study findings', *Journal of Community Psychology*, 47(4), pp. 712–726. 10.1002/jcop.22148

Thompson, G. (2017) 'Long-term perspectives of family quality of life following music therapy with young children on the autism spectrum: A phenomenological study', *Journal of Music Therapy*, 54(4), pp. 432–459. 10.1093/jmt/thx013

Thompson, G. and McFerran, K. (2015) '"We've got a special connection": Qualitative analysis of descriptions of change in the parent-child relationship by mothers of young children with autism spectrum disorder', *Nordic Journal of Music Therapy*, 24(1), pp. 3–26. 10.1080/08098131.2013.858762

Thompson, G., McFerran, K. and Gold, C. (2014) 'Family-centred music therapy to promote social engagement in young children with severe autism spectrum disorder: A randomised controlled study', *Child: Care, Health & Development*, 40(6), pp. 840–852. 10.1111/cch.12121

Thompson, G., Shanahan, E.C. and Gordon, I. (2019) 'The role of music-based parent-child play activities in supporting social engagement with children on the autism spectrum: A content analysis of parent interviews', *Nordic Journal of Music Therapy*, 28(2), pp. 108–130. 10.1080/08098131.2018.1509107

Thompson, M. (2017) *Operation syncopation: Music therapy and autism* https://www.youtube.com/watch?v=gaVtUHOk_RM

Trevarthen, C. and Malloch, S.N. (2000) 'The dance of wellbeing. Defining the musical therapeutic effect', *Nordic Journal of Music Therapy*, 9(2), pp. 3–17.

Tuomi, K., Thompson, G., Gottfried, T. and Ala-Ruona, E. (2021) 'Theoretical perspectives and therapeutic approaches in music therapy with families', *Voices*, 21(2).

Walker, N. (2014) 'What is Autism?', *Neuroqueer: The writings of Dr. Nick Walker*. https://neuroqueer.com/what-is-autism/

Chapter 3

# Perspectives on Social Engagement During Short-Term Dance/Movement Therapy Groups Within an Integrated Special Education Classroom

*Andrea Gleason, Christina Devereaux, and Ryan Matchullis*

## Introduction

Research highlights that creative movement experiences can provide distinct benefits to children with special needs such as building expressive language skills and social functioning (Behrends, Müller and Dziobek, 2012), increasing attentive and task engagement behaviours (Hartshorn et al., 2001; Stamou et al., 2019), and increasing social engagement and play (Nelson et al., 2017). Additionally, several empirical studies have indicated that engaging in the basics of dance/movement can benefit the academic, emotional, and social goals specifically for children within special education classrooms (Hartshorn et al., 2001; Aithal et al., 2021a) as dance provides "layered learning experiences that deepen their repertoire of behaviour and response to the world" (Lorenzo-Lasa, Ideishi, and Ideishi, 2007, p. 25).

Particularly, individuals with an Autism Spectrum Disorder (ASD) may demonstrate variance in "social communication and social interaction across multiple contexts" such as (1) social-emotional reciprocity; (2) nonverbal communicative behaviours used for social interaction; and (3) developing, maintaining, and understanding relationships (American Psychiatric Association, 2013, p. 50) and such challenges can compromise spontaneous social behaviour, social awareness, affect expressivity, prosody, and language development. Porges (2011, p. 220) suggests that "interventions that improve the neural regulation of the social engagement system hypothetically should enhance spontaneous social behaviour, affect regulation, reduce stereotypical behaviours, and improve language skills". Both relational interaction through spontaneous social expressions and body integration through channelling repetitive restrictive behaviours into relationship dances are concepts that dance/movement therapists have been practising with people with ASD and special needs for decades (Scharoun Benson et al., 2014).

DOI: 10.4324/9781003201656-5

The value of dance/movement therapy (DMT) for children with ASD may be due to the nature of dance itself, central to the discipline. A systematic review by DeJesus et al. (2020), for example, examined the influence of dance on negative symptoms for adult individuals with ASD and identified specific aspects embedded within dance through five selected studies that might be contributing factors that influence social communication. Findings emphasised that mirroring, synchronisation, rhythm, and reciprocity had a positive influence on communication, body awareness, behaviour, psychological wellbeing, and social skills. These findings are similar to what Schmais (1985) discussed as the eight *healing processes* embedded within group DMT (synchrony, expression, rhythm, vitalisation, integration, cohesion, education, and symbolism).

In another systematic review (Morris et al., 2021), the effectiveness of mirroring and engagement in rhythm-based interventions were examined to target social communication skills in children diagnosed with ASD. Studies included in the review utilised a variety of outcome measures, including eye gaze, joint attention, and other social behaviours towards the adult. The findings from this review suggested positive effects came from the mirroring and rhythm techniques independently and outside the realm of DMT, suggesting that these might be used effectively to increase communication skills and social development.

In a recent crossover design study (Aithal et al., 2021b), the effects of DMT on children with ASD were investigated by using the Social Communication Questionnaire (SCQ), and Strengths and Difficulties Questionnaire (SDQ) from parents' and teachers' perspectives respectively. The change in the scores from pre- to post-intervention were significantly greater in the DMT intervention group than in controls, suggesting that regardless of the variation of abilities presented by children with ASD, DMT can be successful in furthering the social communication aspects of the children within a short period.

While it is increasingly being recognised that the inclusion of DMT within a classroom setting can provide a healthy outlet for the expression of feelings, collaboration among classroom educators provides valuable information about perceived contributions towards social communication developments. Only a few studies have begun to examine this. Meekums (2008) conducted a pragmatic mixed-methods pilot study of teacher perceptions regarding school-based DMT sessions for six children aged four to seven in a primary school. Data were collected on teachers' perceptions relating to teacher-identified goals, and on movement metaphors reported in the therapist's notes. Results suggested a link between metaphors identified and positive teacher-rated outcomes in areas relating to self-esteem, emotional expression and regulation, and social functioning. Meekums (2008) also indicated that while direct causal links could not be identified due to the uncontrolled design, they could be inferred through qualitative teacher-feedback.

In a qualitative study examining 13 educators' perceptions of the inclusion of DMT within special education classrooms with children diagnosed with ASD and other conditions in the United States, findings emphasised an overall perceived value for the use of DMT to assist the children in gaining focus, modulating energy, and supporting healthy social engagement skills (Devereaux, 2017). Given that multidisciplinary early intervention can support social skill development for children with ASD and other special needs, this study was designed to explore classroom staff reports about DMT's influence on social engagement within early intervention classrooms.

## Study Approach

This study applied a qualitative approach to investigate staff perceptions answering the following research questions: how does participation in the short-term structured group DMT influence social engagement with children within the early intervention classroom? Based on staff experiences, what might be the contributing factors in the DMT sessions that influenced social engagement?

### Procedure and Participants

Dance/movement therapy (DMT) sessions occurred across 38 preschool/kindergarten classes in a specialised school setting with children diagnosed with ASD as well as children with other identified diverse learning needs in Alberta, Canada. Sessions were 20 minutes in duration and held once per week for four to five consecutive weeks. A total of 470 children were enrolled in these classes, with 426 of these children receiving education coding for early intervention support. 164 of these children were coded as having a severe speech and language delay, 228 of the children had education coding for diagnoses such as ASD, global development delay, cerebral palsy, brain injury and Tourette's syndrome. Seven of the children had education coding categorising them as having two or more non-associated moderate to severe cognitive and/or physical disabilities classifying their functioning as severe to profound including diagnoses such as Down's syndrome. Two of the children were classified as having severe emotional/behavioural disabilities, and 25 of the children were classified as having a mild/moderate disability.

In the first week of DMT sessions, the classroom staff were given a 30-minute training session which introduced DMT, including target areas such as emotional expression, regulation and specific reference to 'power posing' to describe the relationship between simple changes of movement (posture change) and self-perception (Carney, Cuddy and Yap, 2010). The training also included the goals of the DMT groups, (supporting self-awareness, shared attention and social connectivity) and described the classroom staff's role in the DMT groups and how they could support the children's participation and enjoyment of the DMT sessions (connecting through movement, modelling the activities, and providing general behavioural support). The training concluded with a description of how the groups would be contributing to individualised programme goals such as impulse control, following adult direction, and participating in structured activities. After each four-to-five-week DMT intervention, semi-structured focus groups were conducted with the classroom team, which included a classroom teacher and up to four classroom staff who had participated in the DMT sessions. Focus groups occurred between one week to five weeks after the intervention was completed. While the exact number of participants was not recorded, an estimated 50%–75% of 83 invited participants took part in the focus groups. Staff were informed that their responses were voluntary, private, and de-identified, and that there were no administrative or other pressures to respond to questions.

### Overall Structure of Each DMT Group

Each group began in a circle formation and followed a similar structure of a warm-up, theme development, and closure (Levy, 2005). However, sessions were modified as necessary based on the need level of the group. The warm-up was an opportunity not only for physical warming of the body and building self-awareness, but also to establish a sense of group unity and comfort. The facilitator guided structured movement activities that focused on encouraging body awareness by tapping and labelling of body parts, exploring movements on different axes and levels, as well as expansion and contraction movements. The use of a ritual "hello" greeting song with accompanying movements provided opportunities for individual expression and prepared them to relate to others.

Next, during the theme development portion, a strong emphasis was placed upon motor development, joining together, and building connections with others on a movement level (moving closer together, reaching towards each other). This varied from session to session but usually involved group activities through synchronistic rhythm, mirroring movement, the use of tactile props to engage the sensory-motor, and structured social games (such as freeze dance, follow the leader, or moving around the room in single file on an imaginary train). These activities provided opportunities for imitation, joint attention, communication, sharing space, and cooperation.

During the closing portion of the session, the primary goal was to regulate the body and integrate their movement experiences before returning to their classroom activities and structure. The use of music, tactile tools like scarves, slower movement experiences, or guided relaxation and breathing exercises supported this process.

## Focus Groups

Classroom staff perceptions of children's social engagement during the DMT sessions were gathered post-DMT-intervention in a focus group structure. The semi-structured questions asked for relevant observations during DMT groups related to perceived changes in social skills and social connectedness, and arousal/focus. The classroom staff were asked questions such as "What observations or changes did you notice in the children's social skills?" and "What observations or changes did you notice in the children's social connectedness?" General questions were also brought forward such as "How were the groups useful?" and providing space for further comments at the end of the group. The focus groups were conducted by a school psychologist not affiliated or connected with the facilitation of the groups to minimise demand characteristics. Discussions were short, lasting a maximum of 15 minutes.

## Data Analysis

Focus group interviews were recorded through hand transcription by the interviewer (3rd author) noting staff comments for each question. Each comment was systematically coded separately by two different coders using descriptive methods (Saldaña, 2009). In the first cycle, each coder separately used a colour-coded descriptive method where significant descriptive statements were assigned a category, or "meaning unit". The meaning units were then examined side by side. The second round of coding consisted of refining the descriptive statement by using "a word or short phrase that assigned a summative attribute ... for a portion of language-based data" (Saldaña, 2009, p. 3) where the meaning units were clustered into a series of organised themes capturing the essence of the reoccurring categories. Because both coders were dance/movement therapists and had individual relationships with the material, some natural bias and desire for a positive outcome existed. As an attempt to set them aside, validation strategies were employed to prevent biases including reflexivity and bracketing (Creswell and Miller, 2000). The coders did not consult upon the data until after the first round of systematic coding and engaged in prolonged engagement with a thorough reading and re-reading of the interview data across multiple weeks.

## Findings

The classroom staff had been employed with the school for an average of 5.6 years, and ranged in age from 18 to 64 years, (mean = 38). 20 of these participants completed an anonymous survey regarding their identified ethnicity. Figure 3.1 shows that 56.5% of participants were European/Caucasian/White (N = 12); this is broadly similar to the wider demographics of the student body. Six participants (28.5%) described their

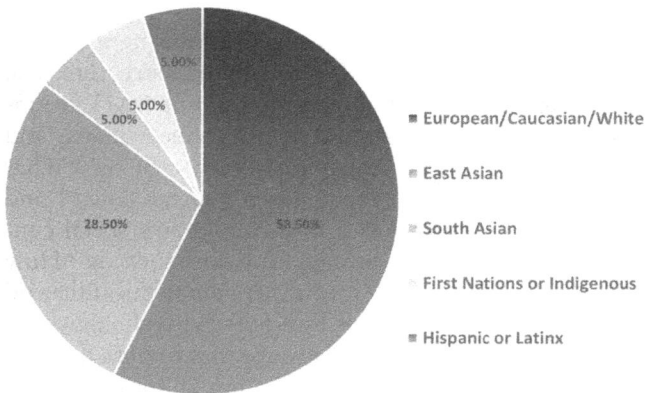

*Figure 3.1* Ethnicity of participants

ethnic background as East Asian. One participant (28.5%) described their ethnic background as South Asian. One participant (5%) described their ethnic background as Hispanic/Latinx. Finally, one participant (5%) described their ethnic background as First Nations or Indigenous.

## Demonstration of Social Engagement

Responses from focus groups identified two overarching themes of observed social engagement across 31 meaning units. Operational definitions of social engagement were drawn from descriptions by *The Social Responsiveness Scale, Second Edition* (SRS-2; Constantino 2012), a screening instrument used to assess autistic spectrum symptoms quantitatively. Relevant to this study, however, the SRS-2 provides descriptive definitions specifically relevant to the research question to further define intervention subscales of social engagement: (1) *social communication* (described as expressive communication categorised by "motoric" aspects of reciprocal social behaviour) and *social motivation* (the extent to which the child is generally motivated to engage in social-interpersonal behaviour including elements of social anxiety, inhibition, and empathic orientation). A second cluster thematic factors relevant to perceived contributions to these social engagement behaviours during the DMT interventions will follow.

### Theme 1: Social communication

Participants described 17 meaning units reflecting three areas of social communication behaviours from the children. These included specific expressive greeting gestures and social actions that were "motoric" aspects of reciprocal social behaviour (eye contact/gaze; greetings/social action; and physical proximity closeness) as discussed below.

## EYE CONTACT/EYE GAZE

Participants reported changes in eye contact. Additionally, accounts of children focusing on the leader with strong eye contact that these participants noted as an indicator in social communication. For example, "One child seemed to have more eye gaze during group" and "There was a social intention never seen before with one female child - went to a person, put her hands out, made eye contact – usually she doesn't acknowledge others at all". Another participant indicated, "children were pretty good at looking at the leader, focusing on directions". While thematically participants perceived eye contact and gaze as an indicator of social communication, cultural considerations regarding the perception of eye contact as a social indicator needs to be cautiously considered.

## GESTURES GREETINGS/SOCIAL ACTION

Participants described particular motoric actions that appeared to reflect social greetings/actions towards others. For example, "Children.. talk to each other, wave hello to each other. And another example, "One of the children has been interested in holding hands with his peers when he is participating in the group". Participants noted the quality of engagement reflecting social actions such as "Participated ... with a smile and a giggle".

## PHYSICAL PROXIMITY/CLOSENESS

Other participants noted adjustments in physical proximity/closeness in space. For example, "When the children get close in the circle, [they] talk to each other, wave hello to each other". One teacher reported that a student "started the group at the end/side of the room, then kept coming closer and closer to me as sessions went on," suggesting that the change in proximity could be indicating a social communication.

### Theme 2: Social Motivation

Social motivation was identified via 13 meaning units describing self-initiating behaviours both individually with peers/adults and generally across the whole group.

## INDIVIDUAL OBSERVATIONS

Several noted behaviours distinct to specific individual children such as an increase in initiating social connections such as "talk[ing] to each other, wav[ing] hello to each other". One staff reported "one [child] started to join a new peer group, imitate actions, and taught [these actions] to classmates". Another reported "one boy seemed not engaged, then started to say 'hello' in the classroom … " And another indicated, "there was social intention never seen before with one female child. She went to a person, put her hands out, and made eye contact. Usually, she doesn't acknowledge others at all".

GROUP-AS-A-WHOLE OBSERVATIONS

Other recognitions of social motivation addressed interactions as the group-as-a-whole. For example, "children seemed generally more engaged and were more engaged with other kids too" and "some were seen to engage much more by the end of the group".

## Contributing Factors Influencing Social Engagement

Five themes emerged within the analysis of the focus group data with the classroom staff that suggested contributing factors within the DMT sessions that may influence social engagement: (1) adaptable and person-centred approaches; (2) novelty; (3) balance in the use of structure and repetition; (4) use of supportive tools; and (5) state regulation of participants as discussed in more detail below.

### Theme 1: Adaptable and Person-Centred Approaches

Allowing the children to "participate in their own way and at their own pace" through adaptable, person-centred approaches was a commonly identified theme. For example, "the group was conducted with developmentally appropriate language and pace" and the facilitator "adapted well to [the children's] needs," "mirror[ed] children and follow[ed] their lead". This supported inclusivity and choice: "kids in wheelchairs or equipment were able to participate, and the group adapted to them," and children were given the "opportunity to lead the movement choices".

### Theme 2: Novelty

Another recurring theme focused on the novelty of the DMT groups (i.e., it was a "special activity," "new experience," "something different") which appeared to have an impact on social engagement. For example, "due to (the DMT group) being novel they really engaged … especially many that wouldn't normally". Another participant noted that this novelty emphasised "new expectations and directions as well as a new routine". For some, there was awareness that over time, the sense of novelty "had worn off" and that engaging in "more novel actions and activities" would be useful. Emphasis was also placed on the role of the facilitator as a "fresh face" or "having a new person teaching/leading the activity".

### Theme 3: Balance in the Use of Structure and Repetition

There were recurring reports that the balance and repetition within the overall session, the content, and the physical structure within the DMT groups were contributing factors toward social engagement. Participants referred to the pace (e.g., "starting slow ... seems to benefit the children"; "sometimes the "cooldown" felt rushed") and the session sequence (e.g., "[the children] benefit from the structure: beginning, middle and end. It helps them anticipate what will happen"). They also questioned whether the activities were "too difficult" or "overly structured," or how "repetition helped with focus". Last, it was noted that the physical structure of the sessions was also an important contributing factor (e.g., variations of the circle formation; group size; duration of the session in time and frequency).

### Theme 4: Use of Supportive Tools

The variety of DMT tools used in the sessions influenced social engagement by either supporting or inhibiting needs. Specifically noted were auditory, visual, or tactile tools like music and scarves that children were "drawn to and liked". These encouraged the children "to dance together" or helped them in "calming ... at the end". These sensory-focused tools worked better than more abstract imagery (e.g., "sleeping dust") that may be more challenging for the children to connect with.

### Theme 5: Regulation of Participants

A common pattern of a change in energy was observed. Sessions began with "very high arousal"; some of the initial activities "got some of the kids fired up". However, "by the end, [the]children always seemed more calm [sic]," they were able to "come down". One respondent placed value on the groups offering different "types of energy". Classroom staff reflected that they perceived a calmer state of regulation in the children towards the end of the group which likely influenced social engagement. This will be discussed further in the following section.

## Discussion

Contributing factors to social engagement, as discussed in the results, were primarily influenced by intentional approaches driven by practitioner choice and presence (e.g. adaptable and person-centred approaches, novelty, balance in the use of structure and repetition, and the use of supportive tools).

This suggests that a person-centred perspective provides a unique and natural opportunity to support social motivation and communication, and is commensurate with other research which reflects that a person-centred approach might support children in "building or initiating social relations on their own" (Aithal et al., 2021a, p. 12). The themes also punctuate the essential bi-directional nature of the social engagement system and the value of co-regulation between facilitator and child. We can infer that when the dance/movement therapist adapted to the need level of the individual or group, the children responded in a way that communicated their level of readiness for social engagement, reflecting their state of regulation.

Assuming that extrinsic factors strongly influence the development of communication and relationships, it is vital to focus on approaches that address the social complexities of ASD. That classroom staff valued the emphasis on a person-centred/individualised approach is in line with Morris et al. (2021) who indicate that dance is a medium that "encourages an inclusive environment, enabling any child, irrespective of their capabilities, to be expressive in a physical and nonverbal manner" (2). A notable extrinsic factor is that the children participating in the group were heterogeneous in their diagnoses and areas of needs and strengths. Therefore, children with social challenges, such as those with ASD, were provided with access to peer models who demonstrated social motivation and communication.

### Regulation: A Calm Mind Supports Social Connections

Previous research emphasised that a regulated state can promote a child's ability to engage socially and to connect with others with the absence of, or diminished sense of a flight/flight/freeze defensive strategies within social interactions (Porges, 2011). This might indicate that body-based interventions specifically can support regulatory mechanisms that impact social engagement. Within theme 5, common discussions highlighted that the children demonstrated a calmer mood at the end of the session. It seems possible that regulatory mechanisms would have provided increased opportunities for learning new social skills, and/or tolerating social pressures.

An additional focus within the discussion group seemed to highlight the importance of co-regulation between classroom staff and the DMT facilitator. Within the focus groups, some classroom staff reflected that the DMT groups provided "increased knowledge of the body and body awareness over time" and referenced its mutual benefit for the staff: "Movement group[s] benefits the teachers, CDFs too: [It] gets them moving, mak[ing] them more mindful," and "[It] feels good to stretch your body". These comments reflect the importance of the support staff playing a co-regulatory role which impacts the social engagement of the children. In addition, perhaps as reported in previous research (Devereaux, 2017), the process of DMT from beginning to end may have a regulating effect for both staff and students.

The classroom teams also noted that understanding their roles and responsibilities influenced their engagement in the groups. This might suggest that the level of regulation and social engagement within the children may have been influenced by reciprocal social communication among support team members as well as the leaders. Further research could focus on deepening the understanding of the intricacies of the connection between social engagement and regulation.

## Implications for Clinical Practice

### A DMT Perspective into the Classroom

The outcomes of the study, while not definitive, still offer several implications for practitioners, educators, and administrators in early childhood settings serving young children with ASD. As suggested by Morris et al. (2021), therapeutic elements commonly used in DMT, such as rhythm and mirroring, could play an effective role in an educational environment. In addition to the co-regulatory function of a person-centred approach, other identified themes from the findings suggest that there are elements of DMT that could be considered for classroom engagement. For example, new structures, including the physical structure of the room, can support the environment for social engagement. In many special education programmes, children sit in an audience format during structured learning time. Instead, the teacher might have the children sit in a circle, providing them with the opportunity to observe and respond to their peers. In addition, social routines could be incorporated into activities to provide regular opportunities for conventional social communication. Similar to other research findings noting the importance of the selection of "motivating materials," this study also amplifies how supportive tools can be generalised to various activities with young children, helping them to share attention and to increase social motivation (Nelson et al., 2017, p. 182). Such motivating materials can also offer tangible opportunities for shared attention and enjoyment. Finally, it appears that maintaining a sense of novelty in classroom activities supports the children to remain interested and engaged. DMT practitioners can also consider the aspect of novelty which may support engagement, while also emphasising the importance of structure and aspects of repetition within the group. Taking a person-centred approach allows for the children to have a "movement voice" and ensures that the practitioner is responding to the needs of the group, based on what is happening within that group dynamic and within each environment.

## Limitations of the Study

Limiting factors were present within the focus groups. The discussions were held at times that the classroom staff would be available, often five to fifteen minutes during a lunch break or at the end of the day. Participation was also voluntary and at times restricted by other tasks that needed to be completed in the classroom. In addition, since the focus groups were held retrospectively, responses were often generalised with limited specific comment. It is possible that this was due to the timing of the interviews within the school day. It also appeared more challenging for the participants to recall enough details from a few weeks back, limiting their capacity to expand on their responses.

An additional limitation was the lack of consistent demographic information from the participants. While participants were able to report on their age, racial, and ethnic identities, this data was not captured at the time of the initial focus groups; instead, it was done, retrospectively. Thus, the data gathered reflects approximately 60% of the participants. Those who identified their race/ethnicity were white/European identified participants. The limited diverse representation among respondents challenges the broader perspectives and cultural considerations of social communication and social motivation. Future studies could examine these distinctions more intentionally.

### Suggestions for Future Research

The results of this study invite several suggestions for research specific to the principles of dance and DMT that may influence social engagement of young children with ASD in inclusive preschool classrooms. Future designs could examine pre-and post-qualitative or quantitative measures from the participating classroom staff, perhaps assigning a staff person to a specific child. Additionally, qualitative data could be gathered from classroom staff immediately after each session or during the intervention, instead of using retrospective focus groups. Further, opportunities could be created for the child participants to also reflect on their experiences within the DMT intervention. As discussed by Aithal et al. (2021a), a common pattern within child-focused research is to ask for feedback from parents and teachers, and the voices of the children are not necessarily reflected. Future studies could strive to empower children through a person-centred approach to identify their own perceptions of their experiences within DMT interventions.

### References

Aithal, S., Moula, Z., Karkou, V., Karaminis, T., Powell, J. and Makris, S. (2021a) 'A systematic review of the contribution of dance movement psychotherapy towards the well-being of children with autism spectrum disorders', *Frontiers in Psychology*, 12, p. 719673. Available at: 10.3389/fpsyg.2021.719673.

Aithal, S., Karkou, V., Makris, S., Karaminis, T., and Powell, J. (2021b) 'A dance movement psychotherapy intervention for the wellbeing of children with an autism spectrum disorder: A pilot intervention study', *Frontiers in Psychology*, 12, p. 588418. Available at: 10.3389/fpsyg.2021.583418.

Association, A.P. (2013) *Diagnostic and statistical manual of mental disorders, Fifth Edition*. 5th edition. Washington, D.C.: American Psychiatric Publishing.

Behrends, A., Müller, S. and Dziobek, I. (2012) 'Moving in and out of synchrony: A concept for a new intervention fostering empathy through interactional movement and dance', *The Arts in Psychotherapy*, 39(2), pp. 107–116. Available at: 10.1016/j.aip.2012.02.003.

Carney, D.R., Cuddy, A.J.C. and Yap, A.J. (2010) 'Power posing: Brief nonverbal displays affect neuroendocrine levels and risk tolerance', *Psychological Science*, 21(10), pp. 1363–1368. Available at: 10.1177/0956797610383437.

Constantino, J.N. (2012) *(SRS$^{TM}$-2) Social Responsiveness Scale, Second edition*. Available at: https://www.wpspublish.com/srs-2-social-responsiveness-scale-second-edition (Accessed: 26 August 2022).

Creswell, J.W. and Miller, D.L. (2000) 'Determining validity in qualitative inquiry', *Theory Into Practice*, 39(3), pp. 124–130. Available at: 10.1207/s15430421tip3903_2.

Devereaux, C. (2017) 'Educator perceptions of dance/movement therapy in the special education classroom', *Body, Movement and Dance in Psychotherapy*, 12(1), pp. 50–65. Available at: 10.1080/17432979.2016.1238011.

DeJesus, B.M., Oliveira, R.C., de Carvalho, F.O., de Jesus Mari, J., Arida, R.M., and Teixeira-Machado, L. (2020) Dance promotes positive benefits for negative symptoms in autism spectrum disorder (ASD): A systematic review. *Complementary Therapies in Medicine*, 49, p. 102299. Available at: 10.1016/j.ctim.2020.102299.

Hartshorn, K., Olds, L., Field, T., Delage, J., Cullen, C. and Escalona, A. (2001) 'Creative movement therapy benefits children with autism', *Early Child Development and Care*, 166(1), pp. 1–5. Available at: 10.1080/0300443011660101.

Levy, F.J. (2005) *Dance movement therapy: a healing art*. 2nd rev. ed. Reston, VA: National Dance Association an Association of the American Alliance for Health, Physical Education, Recreation, and Dance. Available at: http://catdir.loc.gov/catdir/toc/fy0706/88138513.html (Accessed: 26 August 2022).

Lorenzo-Lasa, R., Ideishi, R.I. and Ideishi, S.K. (2007) 'Facilitating preschool learning and movement through dance', *Early Childhood Education Journal*, 35(1), pp. 25–31. Available at: 10.1007/s10643-007-0172-9.

Meekums, B. (2008) 'Developing emotional literacy through individual dance movement therapy: A pilot study', *Emotional and Behavioural Difficulties*, 13(2), pp. 95–110. Available at: 10.1080/13632750802027614.

Morris, P., Hope, E., Foulsham, T. and Mills, J.P. (2021) 'The effectiveness of mirroring- and rhythm-based interventions for children with autism spectrum disorder: A systematic review', *Review Journal of Autism and Developmental Disorders*, 8(4), pp. 541–561. Available at: 10.1007/s40489-021-00236-z.

Nelson, C., Paul, K., Johnston, S.S. and Kidder, J.E. (2017) 'Use of a creative dance intervention package to increase social engagement and play complexity of young children with autism spectrum disorder', *Education and Training in Autism and Developmental Disabilities*, 52(2), pp. 170–185.

Porges, S.W. (2011) *The Polyvagal Theory: Neurophysiological Foundations of Emotions, Attachment, Communication, and Self-regulation*. 1st edn. W. W. Norton & Company.

Saldaña, J. (2009) *The coding manual for qualitative researchers.* Los Angeles, CA: Sage.

Scharoun Benson, S., Luymes, N., Bryden, P. and Fletcher, P. (2014) 'Dance/movement therapy as an intervention for children with autism spectrum disorders', *American Journal of Dance Therapy*, 36. Available at: 10.1007/s10465-014-91 79-0.

Schmais, C. (1985) 'Healing processes in group dance therapy', *American Journal of Dance Therapy*, 8(1), pp. 17–36. Available at: 10.1007/BF02251439.

Stamou, A., Bonneville-Roussy, A., Ockelford, A. and Terzi, L. (2019) 'The effectiveness of a music and dance program on the task engagement and inclusion of young pupils on the autism spectrum', *Music & Science*, 2, p. 205920431988185. Available at: 10.1177/2059204319881852.

Chapter 4

# Practical Implications of the Sensory-Based Relational Art Therapy Approach

*Huma Durrani*

## Introduction

Approximately 96% of children with an autism spectrum disorder (ASD) have issues with sensory integration across multiple domains (Marco et al., 2011) namely: visual, auditory, kinaesthetic, taste, smell, vestibular (sense of movement) and proprioception (sense of body in space). Sensory Integration Dysfunction (SID) is cited as one of the primary causes of dysregulation and high anxiety in children who may retreat into a shell to protect themselves from undesirable input which can have implications for healthy attachment formation (Wing, 1996; Rutgers et al., 2007).

Sensory-Based Relational Art Therapy Approach (S-BRATA) is a framework that addresses SID and attachment issues in children with ASD. It evolved out of the case studies with Teo, Raj and Alex, three boys with ASD with considerable SID. Generated through grounded theory methodology, S-BRATA consists of seven themes and several sub-themes. In this chapter, the model is examined briefly, highlighting the practical implications for therapists. The therapist is positioned as an attachment figure for the highly anxious child who may have had a less than optimal attachment experience with their caregiver due to sensory issues.

### Sensory Integration Dysfunction and Attachment Patterns in Children with ASD

Most therapeutic interventions for children with ASD target the teaching of skills and behaviour modification. While it is important to address these aspects of the child's development, it is equally significant to attend to their emotional needs which often take a backseat to behavioural objectives. A secure attachment pattern has short and long-term implications for the healthy emotional and developmental trajectory of a child. Securely attached children are likely to be more confident, resilient and better regulated than those with insecure attachment patterns (Bowlby as cited in Sroufe et al., 1999).

DOI: 10.4324/9781003201656-6

Table 4.1 Commonly used terms in sensory processing (Durrani, 2021)

| Hyper-responsiveness | Over-reaction to stimuli, examples include aversion to touch and texture such as labels on clothes, dislike of hugs, refusal to walk barefoot on grass, awareness of smells and sounds that may lead to sensory overload. |
| --- | --- |
| Hypo-responsiveness or sensory gating | Under-reaction to stimuli, for example, diminished response to extremely hot and cold surfaces, disengagement from the environment, not responding to the name being called etc. |
| Sensory seeking | Seeking extreme stimulation, for example, enjoy rough play, touching and sniffing objects, excessive fidgeting, swinging etc. |
| Sensory defensive | Negative reaction to sensory input. The child is hyper-responsive to sensory stimuli and protects themselves through negative reactions. |
| Sensory avoidant | Resistance to interact with the environment due to over-response to sensory stimuli. |

The rationale underpinning the intervention involving Teo, Raj and Alex, the children included in this study, is that children with ASD and comorbid SID have a high chance of impaired attachment due to their challenges in processing sensory input from the environment (Marco et al., 2011; Rutgers et al., 2007). As presented in Table 4.1, SID can manifest as hyper and hypo-sensitivities across multiple sensory domains that may lead to high anxiety in children on the spectrum as they may withdraw from their surroundings as a protective mechanism (Marco et al., 2011). Consequently, attachment behaviours that are rooted in sensory perceptions such as touch, gaze, vocalisations and gestures may be hampered between caregiver and child due to these differences in sensory processing (van der Kolk, 2014).

The importance of supporting a child to develop secure attachments cannot be over-emphasised especially since insecure attachment patterns can be replaced by new ones presenting an opportunity for amelioration. Consequently, an approach such as art therapy, that can address both SID and attachment concurrently is fitting due to its multi-sensory nature and relational context (Durrani, 2019).

## Study Approach

S-BRATA is a clinically tested framework generated through grounded methodology based on the three case studies of Teo, Raj and Alex. I chose the boys for the study through purposive sampling, based on the criteria of a diagnosis of ASD and comorbid SID. I used closed Facebook groups to connect with caregivers in Singapore and subsequently assessed the suitability of the children for the study through a preliminary interview with the caregivers and an informal observation of the boys' behaviour in my art therapy studio.

The data for the study was generated from 12 forty-five-minute sessions, one session per week, with Teo, Raj and Alex. I video recorded each session and made detailed clinical notes. An aggregate video of the 12 sessions with each boy was shown to their caregiver and feedback was received in a post-therapy interview. The three aggregate videos and 36 clinical notes were shared with an art therapist for triangulation purposes.

To generate the framework, I coded the data from the sessions into 36 analytic tables. The key concepts that emerged from the analytic tables were translated into three tables, the data from which was compared and coded for recurrence and relevance. This process led to the generation of the seven themes of the S-BRATA (Figure 4.1).

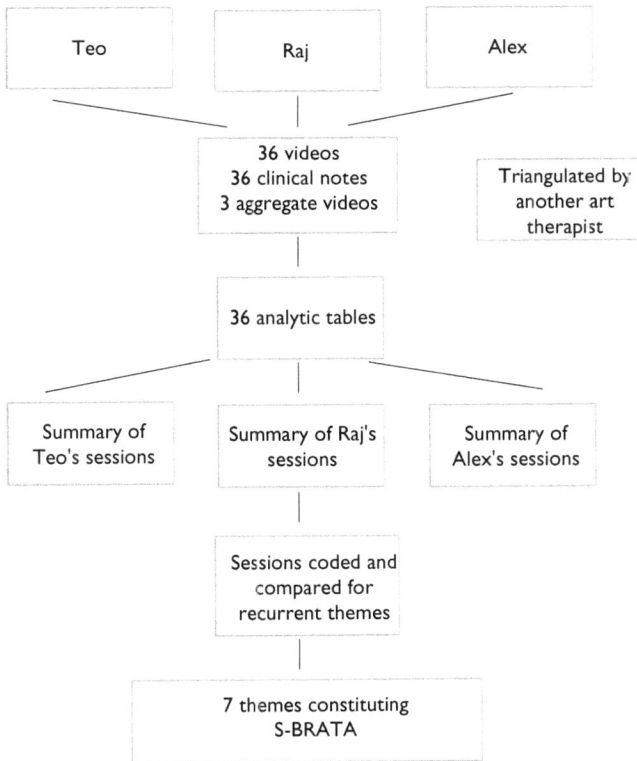

Teo

Raj

Alex

36 videos
36 clinical notes
3 aggregate videos

Triangulated by another art therapist

36 analytic tables

Summary of Teo's sessions

Summary of Raj's sessions

Summary of Alex's sessions

Sessions coded and compared for recurrent themes

7 themes constituting S-BRATA

*Figure 4.1* Methodology (Durrani, 2021)

## Findings and Discussion

### Teo

Five-year-old Teo was verbal but his language was difficult to follow and he kept repeating nursery rhymes. Teo craved touch and movement and had little body awareness, all of which indicated hypo-sensitivities with touch, sense of body in space, balance and movement. He seemed to have no interest in his environment and appeared to be shut down.

### Raj

Seven-year-old Raj had challenges with touch and sense of body in space. He had limited receptive and expressive language and struggled with self-regulation.

### Alex

Alex had age-appropriate language skills at seven years of age but had great difficulty with self-regulation and exhibited separation anxiety from his mother. He was oral seeking, had significant issues with his sense of body in space and a very short attention span.

As indicated in the previous section, the specific model developed from these three children involved seven main themes: (1) sense of safety, (2) working with the child's sensory profile, (3) art materials as entry point for engagement, (4) attachment formation through mirroring and attunement, (5) flexibility in approach, (6) structure and boundaries, and (7) art product not the focus (Durrani, 2021). The seven themes run concurrent to each other and are not necessarily sequential in nature. These themes and associated sub-themes are summarised in Figure 4.2 and further described in this chapter.

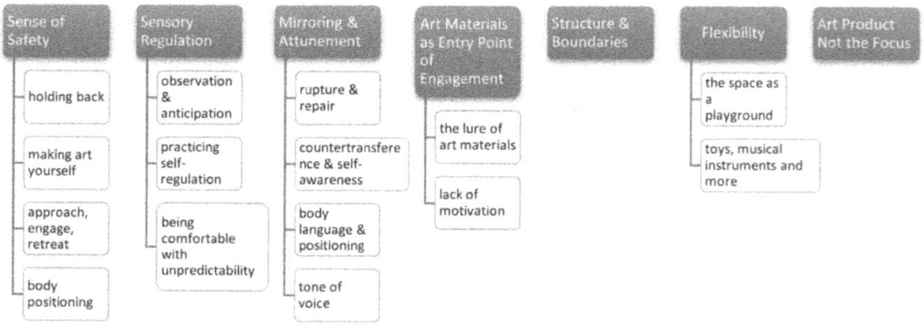

Figure 4.2 The seven themes of the S-BRATA (Durrani, 2021)

## Sense of Safety

I learned from all three boys that it is critical to establish sense of safety for the anxious child, especially one who is new to the therapist. For instance, Teo was mostly shut down from his environment throughout the initial sessions, probably because he did not feel safe. I realised that there was little chance of establishing reciprocity with him if he did not feel secure in my presence. As it happened, once Teo felt safe with me in the room, he began to respond to my overtures and began to open up and pay attention to his surroundings. This might be relevant for the child with ASD whose "sense of safety may be compromised and exacerbated by an incoherent sensory system, difficulty with theory of mind (TOM) and relational and communication difficulties" (Durrani, 2021, 57–58). I attempted to maintain a sense of safety throughout the sessions with Teo, Raj and Alex so that I could create a safe holding space for them. The following sub-themes emanate from the primary theme of safety and illustrate how the latter may be operationalised.

## Holding Back

Holding back refers to the therapist's position of refraining from active engagement with the child so as not to overwhelm them with the expectation of a response. Active engagement means any intrusive or imposing behaviour that may put undue pressure on the child, for instance: repeated name calling; close proximity; commanding attendance or compliance to a plan or activity. I discovered the impact of holding back with Raj who in the initial sessions rejected my advances and dysregulated easily when I approached him persistently. I evidenced a correlation between Raj's increased escalated rigid repetitive behaviours (RRBs), self-stimulatory behaviours and increased level of stress. When highly anxious Raj would continuously run around the room, fidget with pencils or brushes and vocalise loudly, I toned down my eagerness to illicit a response from Raj as I felt the need for space and time before reciprocity could be established. I learned that where the child's level of anxiety may be high due to unfamiliarity with the space and the therapist, any obtrusive attempts at communication may cause an escalation of fear and discomfort.

## Making Art Yourself

While the therapist is in the mode of holding back, they can retreat to a part of the therapy room to make art themselves ideally using materials that will draw the attention of the child. This allows the therapist to allay some of the stress they themselves may be feeling when the child is not responding and it also creates the opportunity for the child to watch the therapist from a safe distance and approach them at their own initiative. For instance, when Teo seemed to not shown any interest in engaging with me, I stood at some distance from him and squirted shaving foam on a tray. The sound of the foam spurting forth from the pressurised container and its fluffy texture, caught Teo's eye who walked up to me to touch the foam. Eventually, I was able to extend our engagement by employing the approach, engage and retreat technique described below.

### Approach, Engage and Retreat

After Teo touched the foam that I spurted in the tray, he quickly lost interest; I retreated to making art myself at a distance from him instead of persistently engaging him. After a few minutes, I attempted to approach Teo to re-engage him and he responded by picking up a blob of foam and fingering it. This pattern of behaviour repeated itself over the next couple of sessions and I learned that when I paced my level of engagement with Teo, spacing out the periods of interaction so as not to overwhelm him, I was able to build his tolerance to proximity with me.

Similar to holding back, the "approach, engage, retreat" technique gives the child time to recoup their resources for relational activity that requires them to exit their comfort zone. Once the child is comfortable with close proximity to the therapist, the latter can focus on extending the cycles of interaction.

### Body Positioning

The therapist's body position refers to where the therapist is standing or seated in relation to the child's eye level. In my sessions with Teo, Raj and Alex I was conscious to adopt an invitational position that was non-threatening with limited eye contact, a tilted head position, with gentle and deliberate movements or gestures (Evans and Dubowski, 2001). If the therapy room is spacious as mine was, it is advisable to use the floor rather than a table and chair for making art oneself as well as with the child. Since Teo lacked body awareness and Raj sought a lot of movement, using a table and chair would have been difficult and possibly restrictive for freedom of movement and accessibility to art materials from all sides.

### Sensory Regulation

In order to form relationships with the child, managing the child's level of anxiety through sensory regulation may be necessary. This requires the therapist to be familiar with the child's sensory profile, their hypo and hyper-sensitivities to various stimuli from the environment (Robledo et al., 2012). This information may be gathered from the child's occupational therapist or their caregiver as well as by observing the child carefully for self-stimulatory or inhibitory behaviours during the sessions.

## Observation and Anticipation

It is important that the therapist remains attentive to the behaviours of the child throughout the session for cues into their regulation status. Armed with prior knowledge of the child's sensory profile, whether from other professionals or the child's family, the therapist can conduct an ongoing assessment of the highs and lows of the child's emotional state which is closely linked to their sensory needs. Hence, keen observation of escalation or reduction in RRB's and self-stimulatory behaviours (e.g., vocalisations, gestures, hand flapping, biting and rocking) is a source of important information to the therapist. I conducted sessions with Teo, Raj and Alex maintaining an anticipatory stance, cognisant of their responses towards certain materials and activities. For example, Alex tended to dysregulate with paint and would get very excited; hence, I monitored its use with him. I noted that playdough seemed to ground Teo; this was evidenced by a reduction of vocalisations and movement. Raj's responses were erratic and at times I was thrown off by his behaviour. Therefore, I often went with the flow and experimented with different art materials and gauged Raj's reaction.

## Practising Self-Regulation

The sensory highs and lows present a great opportunity for practicing self-regulation within the session. The inherent qualities of art materials (discussed later), especially come in handy when inducing cycles of arousal and relaxation. With repeated cycles children learn to internalise the concept of self-regulation by attuning to the body's ability to calm itself down. With Alex, switching between a modulating activity such as pounding, rolling or pinching with playdough followed by a high arousal interaction with a fluid and emotive material such as paint generated a rise and fall in his sensory and emotional responses. Similarly, with Teo, alternating between foam and play dough induced a state of high and low arousal respectively.

## Being Comfortable with Unpredictability

Not only does the therapist have to be fully aware of the variability of a child's sensory profile, they also need to be prepared for any volatility that may result from implicit and explicit factors such as stress, change of routine, environmental and emotional triggers, and so on. A child who has a positive response to a particular art material one day may react negatively to the same on another day. For example, in one session Alex, who usually responded well to kinetic sand-based activities, dysregulated unsuspectingly while engaging with it. I was confounded by his unpredictable reaction not knowing that before coming to the session he had a difficult day at school and was inclined to test my limits in the session. I responded to Alex with support and consistent boundaries. I learned from him that what a child needs from the therapist is the security of a base that they can return to for validation and acceptance; a platform from which they can explore, learn and grow.

### Mirroring and Attunement

The concept of mirroring and attunement is best explicated through the nuanced interactions of the mother-child relationship that underpin the attachment relationship (Gallese, 2009; Schore, 2003). The multi-layered reciprocity between the caregiver and child is rooted in explicit attachment behaviours such as touch, gaze, vocalisations and gestures mediated through sensory channels as well as implicit ones such as recognition, anticipation, "awareness of breath, movement, impulses sensation and associative emotions" (Kossak, 2015, p 37).

Since the S-BRATA positions the therapist as an attachment figure, the overarching theme of the framework is empathic resonance between therapist and child. Simply put it can be understood as a moment-to-moment connection felt through the senses and practiced through the actions of the therapist. For example, in order to connect with Teo who was averse to interaction with the outside world due to high anxiety or lack of motivation, I found a way to connect in a non-threatening way. This was done by observing him carefully for behaviours that I could mirror back to him, just like a mother and child duo where the former responds in kind to the latter's smiles or vocalisations. Hence, I joined Teo in singing his nursery rhymes, jumped and ran with him around the room to indicate my desire to communicate at his level. Again, I tried to maintain a sense of safety across all aspects of the intervention as well as an awareness of Teo's sensory sensitivities.

### Rupture and Repair

Similar to the ups and downs in any relationship, the therapist-child relationship may hit a rough patch after an attachment has been formed. This state of upheaval can last for a couple of sessions or even longer and can take the form of oppositional behaviour, tantrums, or not wanting to come for the sessions. This can be extremely disconcerting and stressful for the therapist as well as for the child. At times this rupture may come out of nowhere completely throwing the therapist off who may suddenly feel disconnected and out-of-synch with the child. This happened in one session with Alex: he had a huge melt-down and I ended the session prematurely because of his disruptive behaviour. At that moment I felt that the intervention had hit a roadblock, but I realised later that rupture and repair are part of any attachment relationship. The falling out-of-synch and overriding the storm is where the learning takes place for both the therapist and the child. It is an opportunity to test the strength of the relationship by setting boundaries, pushing limits and letting the child know that despite a breakdown in the relationship, there is a safe holding space with the therapist to which the child can return (Kossak, 2015). In the next session, Alex rebounded as if nothing had happened, and I felt my sense of confidence return. The onus through such an upheaval is on the therapist to maintain a state of equilibrium and trust the process, provided the work on establishing the sense of safety and attuning has been done in earlier sessions.

### Counter-Transference and Self-Awareness

What lies at the core of the theme of mirroring and attunement is the deep visible and invisible connection between therapist and child, with varying shades of physical and emotional interactions. With the interplay of give and take, harmony and disharmony, there are feelings being projected onto the therapist by the child and vice versa (Evans and Dubowski, 2001). The therapist can learn to use these emotional reactions (transference and counter-transference) to their advantage by enhancing emotional responses or channelising them in other directions. For example, when Alex acted in an oppositional way towards me in the session mentioned above, I emulated the role of an attachment figure and imposed boundaries around him, such as a caregiver or parent might do to counter their child's behaviour. I recognised my feelings of love and care towards Alex, as well as irritability and frustration, as caregivers often do. Identifying this as counter-transference enabled me to focus on the goal of the intervention rather than get swayed by the emotion.

This kind of self-awareness requires skill and alertness throughout the session. The therapist can find cues into the relational dynamics between themselves and the child by paying close attention to what is happening inside their body. For example, in some sessions I experienced an escalation of heart rate in reaction to Raj's increased anxiety. At times, my anxiety manifested as a knot in my stomach, tension in the shoulders, and changes in my posture, indicative of the pervading emotion between myself and Raj. With Teo, I felt a softening of my posture and an inclination to use a softer tone of voice, underpinned by a feeling of protectiveness.

### Tone of Voice

Some children like Alex require a higher pitched tone of voice to attend to the therapist including effusive praise and high fives. Others, like Teo, are comfortable with a lower but firm and consistent pitch. It may appear daunting to the therapist to be mindful of so many aspects of the interaction. However, once the therapist is attuned to the child, most of these things fall into place naturally. It is important to go with the flow and enjoy being with the child, since pleasure in reciprocity is what strengthens the bond between the therapist and child.

### Art Materials as Entry Point of Engagement

The wonderful resource that art therapists have in the form of art materials is unparalleled in its variety and applicability. From traditional art materials (such as paint, pencils, crayons, markers and clay) to non-traditional ones (shaving foam, goop/slime, found objects, and so on), the list can be endless. My art therapy room is sufficiently stocked with a variety of materials to cater to a wide range of sensory needs. For children who have an impaired sense of body in space, I have clay, play dough and sand that can be pounded, squeezed and moulded. For tactile-seeking children, paint mixed with glue and sand can be a good motivator to use with hands. For highly anxious children, more restrictive materials like pencils and crayons can be beneficial. Of course, one cannot generalise about which material will serve what purpose, but the point is that during any one session the therapist may need to switch mediums to induce regulation or to keep the child engaged. Art materials are usually the therapist's first point of entry for engagement with the child, as most children are drawn by their multi-sensory qualities. Especially with children who are resistant to relational activity, the art materials can act as a buffer or intermediary.

Some points to consider while setting up the therapy room: (a) protecting the floor with a plastic sheet or other surface sometimes may be necessary to reduce the cleaning process; (b) storing paint in ketchup bottles and cutting the tips of the bottles in varying sizes can control the amount of material dispensed; (c) using washable paint; (d) keeping a good supply of kitchen paper roll and wet wipes; (e) having a collection of small toys, a variety of balls and a couple of musical instruments at hand.

### The Inherent Qualities of Art Materials

Art materials are available in many formulations, colours, textures, smells and consistencies. They can be applied in any number of ways to create multi-dimensional art forms. The multi-sensory nature of art materials lends them unique characteristics that evoke physiological and emotional responses enhanced by the way they are handled, applied or manipulated, through tools or directly by hand, and also by the surfaces that they are used upon which could vary in texture, size and placement (Malchiodi, 2002). For instance, paint, especially tempera and water colour, is a fluid medium that is hard to control and evocative in nature. It tended to cause high arousal in Alex who responded inversely to playdough and kinetic sand, mediums with centring quality that work well for containment and lower excitability.

Similarly, crayons and pastels provided sufficient proprioceptive input to Alex as they required force to be smudged and blended. Foam, on the other hand, caused him to become excitable, due to its light textural qualities. Cutting and pasting was another grounding activity for Alex, and tearing and crushing paper helped channel his anxiety and frustration. Squirting paint from a height from ketchup bottles attracted all three boys to approach me and engage with the art material.

## The Lure of Art Materials

The child who is new to the therapist or enclosed in a shell may hesitate to engage, but they may be open to the lure of familiar or novel art materials. I found that shaving foam often did the trick with Teo and Raj who were drawn to touch it; once they had made that first move, I got the opening to increase our cycles of engagement. From there, I moved on to spreading the foam on a tray or the plastic sheet on the floor, adding paint or sand to it to heighten their motivation to touch and feel the materials. Most children show a preference for a certain material and that can be used to the therapist's advantage as and when the child needs to be motivated or regulated. Teo was almost always drawn to foam and playdough. Raj was harder to motivate, but he too responded favourably to foam as compared to other art materials. I introduced new materials like glass markers and stickers to draw Alex's attention and was able to distract him from an impending tantrum.

## Lack of Motivation

For some children, art materials may not be a big draw and the therapist can struggle with ideas to engage the child, as I did sometimes with Raj. In that case, toys or musical instruments come in handy, as does movement and play such as catch or roll the ball, throwing darts, or netting baskets if the space allows. I played catch in the sessions with all three boys, and I used drums with both Raj and Teo to motivate them.

## Structure and Boundaries

Children with ASD are known to respond well to structure since it lends predictability and order to tasks and the environment in general. Especially where there is a high degree of SID, or psychomotor impairment, our highly sensory world can be a navigational and attentional nightmare for the child with sensory issues. Consequently, most behavioural interventions for children on the spectrum are designed to be highly structured. art therapy, in comparison to the behavioural interventions, may be considered loosely structured and therapists use a combination of directive and non-directive approaches. A non-directive approach is primarily client-led where the therapist focuses on the present and goes with the flow. A directive approach may one based on a pre-determined plan with a series of activities or instructions lined up for the client.

Within the S-BRATA, there is a place for both directive and non-directive approaches since each child has a different set of needs and the therapist has to recognise what works best for whom. Having said that, the principle that underpins the approach is one of forming an attachment with the child by lowering anxiety levels and attuning to them. Consequently, there is a constant interchange of physical and emotional energy which could get stifled by too much structure. Hence, the therapist should follow the lead of the child. However, if the child is not able to handle a very loose structure then there may be no option but to plan the session in advance to avoid an escalation of anxiety. Teo, Raj and Alex guided me to the structure and boundaries they required. For instance, Alex had a very low attention span and a tendency to get bored easily. Therefore, I had to plan a succession of activities before the session to sustain his engagement. I ensured easy access to art materials he enjoyed and could quickly switch from one activity to another, consequently sessions with him were more structured than with Teo and Raj. Setting clear limits was necessary for Alex who had tendency to push boundaries. When Alex started throwing art material in one session and would not stop even after being informed of the consequences, I ended the session even though he did not want to leave.

For each child, the therapist can determine beforehand what might be acceptable and unacceptable behaviours in the session. For example, is smearing paint on the walls a "no" or a "yes" for a child who is resistant to engaging with art materials and has done so for the first time? What is the boundary for a child such as Teo who has little body awareness and walks all over playdough pasting it onto the floor? With regards to oppositional behaviour, to what extent is a tantrum acceptable before the session is cut short? What kind of physical boundaries are acceptable? Should the child be allowed to hug the therapist or sit in their lap as Raj tended to do? Whatever the case, boundaries should be clearly communicated to the child's caregiver beforehand and once established should remain constant so that the child does not get confused or take advantage of them.

## Flexibility

Over the past few decades, art therapy has evolved into a hybrid of different psychological approaches, broadening its scope to include a range of expressive modalities (Rubin, 2016). Therapists can choose to espouse specific orientations or be eclectic in nature. The complex nature of ASD requires constant innovation, adjustment and adaptation to cater to the varied needs of the child, leaving no space for rigidity in the S-BRATA; an open and flexible attitude is required, where the child and therapist are partners and co-creators.

### The Space as a Playground/Toys Musical Instruments and More

If the person of the therapist is the personification of safety, then the art therapy room is the metaphor for security and containment. I visualised my room as a place of comfort and joy, freedom and expression for Teo, Raj and Alex. Teo was able to sit or lie down on the floor to make art, Alex played hide and seek under the table and Raj ran all around the room. All three boys had access to a chair and table, would throw a ball, play with toys, bang drums and retreat quietly to a corner if desired. I moved away from the traditional mode of sitting at the table and making art with the children to what felt like becoming a child myself. I was willing to do whatever it took to enter the boys' worlds. This meant having a lot of cleaning to do afterward, especially if there were handprints on the walls (walls can be painted with washable paint or have a mirror-lined wall on which to use glass markers or paint), paint on the plastic sheets, and shaving foam and slime spread on the table.

My art therapy room is stocked with a range of stimming objects, some play therapy toys, plastic body parts, different types of balls, a plastic tea or dinner set, kinetic sand and tray and a few musical instruments that come in handy for motivation, distraction, and of course play. Activities such as packing plastic moulds with kinetic sand or excavating hidden objects underneath a mound of sand are entertaining and grounding for children like Alex and Teo who seek excessive tactile input.

### Art Product Not the Focus

Throughout the discussion of the themes of the S-BRATA, the focus has been on the process and not the product. The fact is that for children functioning at the stage of sensory and kinaesthetic expression like Teo and Raj the art product does not hold much value; their capacity for reflection on the art product may be impacted due to multiple cognitive and developmental challenges (Durrani, 2021). Hence, the process of engaging with the art materials as a conduit to a relationship with the therapist becomes more important than the art product itself. For children like Alex, who can make representational art or have the capacity for symbolic thinking, the art product can be a source of accomplishment and joy when shared with others as well as used for other therapeutic purposes that may be developmental or psycho-emotional in nature.

### Conclusion

S-BRATA is a preliminary framework that is recommended as a guide for professionals working with children on the spectrum. Although it is presented as an art therapy-based intervention that evolved out of working with children with ASD, it is not limited in its scope to them nor is it for the use of art therapists alone. Because the themes of the S-BRATA are not prescriptive and are inherently flexible, they can be adapted by all professionals using mind-body approaches that are multi-sensory in nature and applied to children with varying psycho-emotional and developmental needs.

Further research and development of the S-BRATA can focus on dyadic sessions with caregiver and child where the therapist can model attachment behaviours for the former through the art making process. Not only will this facilitate the strengthening of the bond between caregiver and child but also it will equip the former with strategies that can be generalised to communication and behaviours outside the therapy room.

## References

Durrani, H. (2019) 'Art therapy's scope to address impaired attachment in children with ASD and comorbid SID', *Art Therapy*, 37(3), pp. 131–138 doi: 10.1080/07421656.2019.1677063

Durrani, H. (2021) *Sensory-based relational art therapy approach. Supporting psycho-emotional needs in children with autism.* New York: Routledge.

Evans, K. and Dubowski, J. (2001) *Art therapy with children on the autistic spectrum.* London, United Kingdom: Jessica Kingsley.

Gallese, V. (2009) 'Mirror neurons, embodied simulation and the neural basis of social identity', *Psychoanalytic Dialogues*, 19(5), pp. 519–536. doi: 10.1080/10481880903231910.

Kossak, S. Mitchell (2015) *Attunement in expressive arts therapy.* Illinois, USA: Charles Thomas. Publishers.

Malchiodi, A. Cathy. (2002) *The soul's palette.* Boston, MA: Shambala.

Marco, J.E., Hinkley, N.B.L., Hill, S.S. and Nagarajan, S.S. (2011) 'Sensory processing in autism: A review of neurophysiological findings'. *Pediatric Research*, 69(5), pp. 48–54.

Robledo, J., Donnellan, M.A. and Strand-Conroy, K. (2012) 'An exploration of sensory and movement differences from the perspective of individuals with autism', *Frontiers in Integrative Neuroscience*, 6(107), pp. 1–13. doi: 10.3389/fnint.2012.00107.

Rubin, A.R. (ed.) (2016) *Approaches to art therapy.* New York, NY: Routledge.

Rutgers, A.H., van Ijzendoorn, M.H., Bakermans-Kranenburg, M.J., Swinkles, S.H., van Daalen, E., Dietz, C. and van Engeland, H. (2007). 'Autism, attachment and parenting: A comparison of children with autism spectrum disorder, mental retardation, language disorder and non-clinical children', *Journal of Abnormal Child Psychology*, 35(5), pp. 859–870. doi: 10.1007/s10802-007-9139-y.

Schore, N. Alan (2003) 'Early relational trauma, disorganized attachment, and the development of a predisposition to violence', in F.M. Solomon and J.D. Siegel (eds.) *Healing attachment, trauma, mind, body and brain.* New York, NY: W.W. Norton & Company, pp. 107–167.

Sroufe, A.L., Carlson, A.E., Levy, K.A. and Egeland, B. (1999) 'Implications of attachment theory for developmental psychopathology', *Development and Psychopathology*, 11(1), pp. 1–13.

van der Kolk, B. (2014) *The body keeps the score.* New York, NY: Penguin Books.

Wing, L. (1996) 'Autistic spectrum disorders', *Bmj*, 312(7027), pp. 327–328.

Chapter 5

# Shine a Light on Autism

Group Dramatherapy with Children Identified
with Autism and Autistic Traits Who
Experience Anxiety

*Emma Ramsden, Sònia Barrachina, Lynn Cedar,
Xavier Fontenille, Deborah Haythorne, and
Jeannie Lewis*

## Introduction

This chapter focuses on the Emotion Stones, an arts-based method and resource which was incorporated into the intervention design of the feasibility study known as Shine a Light on Autism (SaLoA) (see Figure 5.1, The Emotion Stones). This study was conducted in two educational settings with children aged 7–11 by Roundabout, the UK's leading dramatherapy charity, a London-wide service provider since 1985. Roundabout has developed a specialism in working with autistic people in a wide variety of settings over more than three decades and has published aspects of this work (Haythorne and Seymour, 2017). As an experienced team of practitioners, we came to the project with extensive knowledge of the value of group dramatherapy. However, we had wondered how to capture this in order to promote shared practice within the field and contribute to the research discourse. Roundabout secured funding to develop SaLoA, with the research intention to establish whether group dramatherapy is a helpful intervention for autistic children who experience high levels of anxiety and to investigate if group dramatherapy helps to develop emotional vocabulary, express worries and anxieties and create meaningful relationships for increasing social engagement and wellbeing.

Each of the 12 Emotion Stones depicts a different emotion and is designed to enable children to learn, talk about and express feelings (Yellow-door.net, 2021). This resource was incorporated into the overall design and used in each session over a period of 20 weekly group dramatherapy sessions, yielding rich data showing how participants identified and communicated feelings and emotions, and expressed and managed areas of anxiety and worry. Findings from research data are presented in this chapter, accompanied by a selection of participants' artwork.

DOI: 10.4324/9781003201656-7

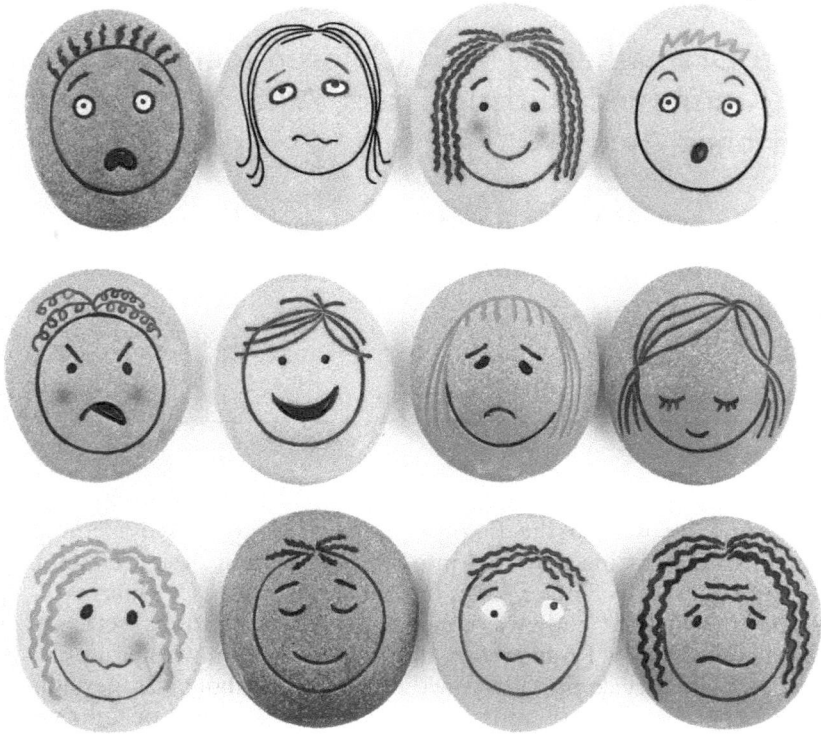

*Figure 5.1* The Emotion Stones (Reproduced with permission from http://www.yellow-door.net)

*Source:* © Yellow Door Emotion Stones (Yellow-door.net, 2021).

As practitioners in the field, anecdotal knowledge suggests that an increasing number of practitioners who work with children and young people are drawing on this resource in their practice, but a survey of current literature shows this to be the first publication to draw on their use, or the use of similar tactile three-dimensional emotional faces, in any dramatherapy setting. However, there is evidence that one-dimensional drawings of emotions and faces have been used outside of the arts therapies in Cognitive Behaviour Therapy (CBT) (Attwood, 2004).

### Roundabout's Ethos

At the heart of SaLoA's design and Roundabout's working ethos is an active investment and belief in client-led practices, with methodologies that enable agency, collaboration and the co-creation of meaning to support wellbeing through children expressing their voices and self-reporting experiences (Jones et al., 2021, chapter 7: 104–127; Ramsden (2017, pp. 61). Roundabout's ethos includes actively holding in mind clients' experiences and their confidentiality with parent/carer involvement and professional input (teachers, therapists, other agencies). At Roundabout, we acknowledge the increasing acceptance of self-identified reporting in educational settings and we embrace self-advocacy and identity-first language (Roundabout Dramatherapy, 2022).

## Autism, Anxiety and Dramatherapy

There is currently a deficit of published research in dramatherapy focusing on anxiety and autism, despite the increased prevalence of anxiety disorders amongst autistic people being well documented in medical literature (Vasa and Mazurek, 2015; Simonoff et al., 2008; Kerns et al., 2014). Van Steensel et al.'s meta-analysis reports nearly 40% of children with an autism diagnosis reaching clinical thresholds for at least one anxiety disorder (2011). For autistic children, generalised and specific types of anxiety can often be exacerbated by, for example, fear of social situations and unexpected changes, and self-imposed pressure to conform in school; these can have a huge impact on a child's ability to maintain wellbeing or function in all areas of daily living including engagement with education (Murin et al., 2016). Diagnosed anxiety disorders and increased levels of anxiety can, for example, lead to sensory sensitivity, difficulties in developing peer relationships, and challenges when engaging with learning. Anxiety can also contribute to negative experiences such as isolation, depression and school refusal.

Resources and psychological interventions for the management of anxiety for autistic people are available (Middletown Centre for Autism, 2020; Nadeau et al., 2011), but very little is written about how dramatherapy can help with this issue. The drive to address this area of unmet need was one of the key factors that led to the design and delivery of this study (Ramsden and Haythorne, 2021). Dramatherapy can be helpful for autistic children, young people and adults, as it supports the development of social skills and the expression of feelings through structured work that can help reduce anxiety (Benbow, 2017, p. 117; Godfrey and Haythorne, 2017, p. 162; Ibid., 2013, p. 21).

This study is rooted in the history of dramatherapy in the UK and work with autistic children from its early developmental stages more than half a century ago (Jennings, 1978; Lindkvist, 1997). Accounts of successful dramatherapy group work are documented in the literature (Jones, 1996; Haythorne, 2012; Dyer, 2017), with outcomes of the group process described as "group members become more fluent with perceiving themselves, perceiving others, perceiving themselves as others and perceiving others as themselves" (Chasen, 2011, p. 261). Of particular note is the reference by the National Autistic Society to the use of structure, cited by Dix (2017, p. 75): "Dramatherapy can make an important contribution to this client group (NAS website; Godfrey and Haythorne, 2013), as it develops social skills through a structured framework, which may reduce anxiety through its use of verbal and nonverbal techniques". SaLoA therefore builds on this work alongside that of Haythorne and Seymour, who note:

> Dramatherapy can reach out to people on the autistic spectrum by recognising differences and individuality, and through a broad range of techniques it can support people to express their feelings and imagination and to develop their communication and social skills.
>
> (Haythorne and Seymour, 2017, p. 9)

## Study Approach

The study took place in schools where Roundabout had long-standing service level agreements. Gatekeeper consent was sought from the schools prior to commencing any aspect of the research. The study received ethical clearance via the Kings College, London (KCL) ethics committee, under the voluntary guidance of a KCL senior lecturer. However, the study was neither in partnership with KCL, nor part of any formal research within the university's portfolio.

Fieldwork for the study was conducted over one academic year (September to July) following the regular flow of the Roundabout model. This consisted of 20 sessions of manualised group dramatherapy delivered to two groups of five children, in two mainstream primary schools both of which had an autism base (a unit which is part of a mainstream provision offering focused educational and pastoral support by specialist teachers and staff). Each of the research groups was facilitated by two dramatherapists.

The ten participants, four female (two Dual Heritage, one Black British, one White British), six male (one Dual Heritage, five White British), met the eligibility criteria in that they were junior school age (7–11 years) with a diagnosis of autism spectrum condition or displaying autistic traits, affected by anxiety, comfortable using verbal language and working in a small group, with no previous experience of dramatherapy. Children who had already received dramatherapy and/or who were presenting with complex needs such as sensory disorders or dual diagnosis, and who were not comfortable using verbal language, formed the exclusion criteria. Pre-, during, post- and three-month follow-up outcome measure interviews were conducted by the lead researcher with children (outside of sessions), parents and teachers, and included an autism and anxiety specific measure (a 21-item rating scale with questions in four anxiety domains: performance anxiety, anxious arousal, uncertainty and separation anxiety) (ASC-ASD, Rogers et al., 2016). The anxiety-specific measure was included to compare pre- and post-outcomes to calculate the effect of treatment.

At the very heart of SaLoA's design is the capacity to utilise therapeutic techniques related to and including opportunities for engaging with story-making (Davidson, 2017, p. 16). This is framed within the 'embodiment-projection-role' (EPR) paradigm developed by dramatherapist Jennings (1993, p. 25) which "charts the dramatic development of children" enabling them to "enter the world of imagination and symbol, the world of dramatic play and drama". Storymaking was one of a number of key areas of SaLoA's design, it is not explored in any detail in this chapter. The theoretical frame focuses on the concepts of children's voice, choice and agency, and draws on earlier work on children as co-researchers of their own therapy (Ramsden and Jones, 2011; Jones et al., 2021). Children chose their own pseudonyms and gave formal assent for the use of their artwork and feedback about their experiences to be drawn on in publications.

The inclusion of the Emotion Stones (a 12-item play-based self-reporting resource) in the overall study design emerged from the idea that autistic people find it hard to read faces and understand social cues and communication (Attwood, 2004). We specifically incorporated this resource because of its potential both as a drama and roleplay activity to explore embodying the faces on the stones and experience them through interoception (connecting with feelings inside the body), and from a sensory aspect, acknowledging the importance of the tacit experience of the feel of the stones and the connection between sensory over-responsivity and anxiety (Green and Ben-Sasson, 2010). The Emotion Stones provided opportunities for the participants to identify and make choices about feelings, share them and listen to selections made by others. Choosing to listen came with a sense of responsibility and agency to make the choice to give the focus to others, fostering connections through identification and difference.

Each session followed a similar structure with one dramatherapist in the lead therapist role, holding the overall structure of the session, and the other as a supporting therapist, who worked alongside the children within the group. The lead and support therapists alternated their roles each week. The session began with a check-in where the children greeted each other and shared the news. This allowed the facilitators to assess individual children's concerns, levels of presenting anxiety and wellbeing, and to observe emerging group themes. This was followed by a warm-up leading toward the main part of the session where the group explored story-making using a variety of dramatherapeutic techniques. The participants were then invited to de-role and move into a process of reflection drawing on the use of the Emotion Stones as a way to appraise their experience. Following the main story-making part of each group dramatherapy session, and before the goodbye and ending, participants were asked to "choose a stone/s that shows how you feel now. Are there any words to go with that?". Built into the session structure was a level of flexibility drawing on the "or something else" principle, which welcomed individual self-expression in each session contained within the overall repetitive structure, and which supported the development of understanding of the idea of intolerance of uncertainty (Boulter et al., 2014). (For more information about SaLoA and to download the 20-session intervention manual please visit https://www.roundaboutdramatherapy.org.uk/.)

### Data Collection and Analysis

Qualitative data were captured by way of session notes with documented therapist observations, verbatim contributions from participants, along with their artwork and choices of Emotion Stones, and were analysed using an inductive thematic analysis approach (Braun and Clarke, 2006). SaLoA yielded 100% data return for children, parents/carers and teachers, and no participant attrition. The delivery of the intervention followed a robust ethical protocol with regard to inviting parents to engage with pre- post- and follow-up meetings to complete outcome measures with the lead researcher, and to attend clinical case meetings with the therapists. This full complement of data return from both children and adults occurred against the backdrop of one school advising that they expected low engagement (if any) from their parents/carers.

## Findings

### Children's Experiences with the Emotion Stones

Qualitative data revealed that the children engaged and invested in attending dramatherapy in a group setting, expressing and exploring feelings, worries and anxieties, developing connections with others and practising social interaction skills, through engagement in story-making.

The Emotion Stones were a successful part of the overall design with the findings showing how relationship-building and the development of social skills through shared engagement in the creative group process was meaningful and empowering for the children. The findings show that as the intervention progressed, increased emotional literacy was present and insights into the children's thinking and feeling emerged in relation to their attending dramatherapy, captured in the words they ascribed to their choices of Emotion Stones on a session-by-session basis. Participants reflected their enjoyment in the familiarity of the session structure and being able to choose Emotion Stones, and they identified that this led them to "being seen" and having choices heard and respected. The next section expands on the findings in relation to the use of Emotion Stones.

Figure 5.2 shows the range of emotional states given to the stones from across the cohort throughout the study. The different words offered by the

Emotional states attributed to each stone across the cohort

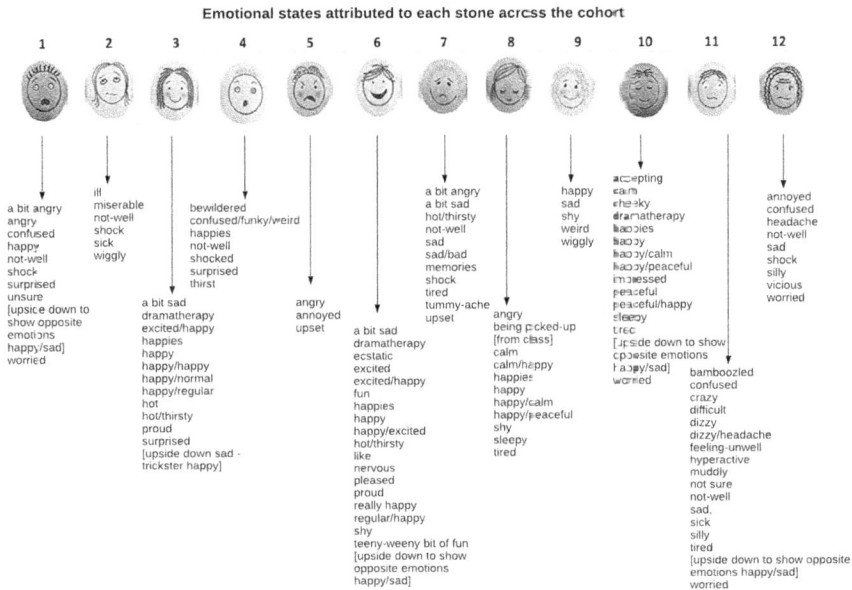

| 1 | 2 | 3 | 4 | 5 | 6 | 7 | 8 | 9 | 10 | 11 | 12 |
|---|---|---|---|---|---|---|---|---|---|---|---|

a bit angry
angry
confused
happy
not-well
shock
surprised
unsure
[upside down to
show opposite
emotions
happy/sad]
worried

ill
miserable
not-well
shock
sick
wiggly

a bit sad
dramatherapy
excited/happy
happies
happy
happy/happy
happy/normal
happy/regular
hot
hot/thirsty
proud
surprised
[upside down sad -
trickster happy]

bewildered
confused/funky/weird
happies
not-well
shocked
surprised
thirst

angry
annoyed
upset

a bit sad
dramatherapy
ecstatic
excited
excited/happy
fun
happies
happy
happy/excited
hot/thirsty
like
nervous
pleased
proud
really happy
regular/happy
shy
teeny-weeny bit of fun
[upside down to show
opposite emotions
happy/sad]

a bit angry
a bit sad
hot/thirsty
not-well
sad
sad/bad
memories
shock
tired
tummy-ache
upset

angry
being picked-up
[from class]
calm
calm/happy
happies
happy
happy/calm
happy/peaceful
shy
sleepy
tired

happy
sad
shy
weird
wiggly

accepting
calm
cheeky
dramatherapy
happies
happy
happy/calm
happy/peaceful
impressed
peaceful
peaceful/happy
sleepy
tree
[upside down to show
opposite emotions
happy/sad]
worried

bamboozled
confused
crazy
difficult
dizzy
dizzy/headache
feeling-unwell
hyperactive
muddly
not sure
not-well
sad,
sick
silly
tired
[upside down to show opposite
emotions happy/sad]
worried

annoyed
confused
headache
not-well
sad
shock
silly
vicious
worried

*Figure 5.2* Emotional states attributed to the stones by participants

children to describe their feelings and experiences amount to more than 125 different terms. One participant added an "upside down" option for some of the selected stones to depict the counter opposite emotion, as by turning the stone upside down, for example with numbers 1, 6 or 10, a smile becomes a sad face and vice versa. For this child, who chose as his pseudonym Gilleus, the changing of a smile into a frown or sad face was a clear way of expressing his conflicting and, at times, ambivalent feelings.

Snow Waffle (participant selected pseudonym; as with all participant names used in this chapter) developed a system of sub-categorising what she referred to as *the happies*. Predominantly using stones 3, 6, 8 and 10, this involved her naming different states of happiness, which included peaceful-happy, excited-happy, very calm-happy, regular-happy and happy-happy. In looking closely at her choices, she consistently reported calm-happy, as well as naming bodily states such as "thirsty" and "hot".

The use of Emotion Stones provided an opportunity for children to create their own emotional language. There was no right or wrong, and over the duration of the fieldwork (20 sessions) children might give a different name to the same stone. The therapists deliberately used feeling words in the sessions to model the language and to support children to think in terms of their emotional states both as themselves and in their character roles chosen during the story-making process at the heart of each session.

What is notable, from the extensive list of feelings and emotional experiences given by the participants, is the awareness that a simple smiley face can hold so many variations and that, generally speaking, participants understood and identified the faces in relation to the resource guide provided with the Emotion Stones (which was not used in the design, as the value of what each child saw in each stone was the focus). Each stone (eg., number 6, the most frequently selected stone) bore multiple connections and subtleties of emotion, demonstrated through the nuanced expression and variations offered. Each participant utilised the Emotion Stones in individual and empowering ways and reflected on their enjoyment of the stones as a way to name their feelings and how good it was to have this opportunity during dramatherapy sessions. Children were supported and challenged to be patient and interested in one another and to respond to the news and ideas other children brought in. This meant an exploration in the group of empathy, theory of mind and mentalising (Fonagy and Allison, 2014) through trying to imagine someone else's experiences.

Making multiple choices of stones was a common feature across the cohort. For example, at the end of session number 15, Jowey, one of the participants in the study, selected stones 3 "happy story", 7 "sad", 5 "angry" and 10 "calm". His selections show the range of experiences contained in a single session and that, as he often did, he chose to reflect chronologically on the session's journey from the story created in the main part of that week's session, through to feeling calm at the session's close. Likewise, another participant in the study, Ginger Kitten, retraced her feelings in session 9 from starting with sadness, moving through anger and into feeling happy at the end. Witnessing other children's feelings also helped children not to feel alone, recognising that others were expressing similar feelings. As well as choosing Emotion Stones, for some children drawing images was an important part of the session's reflection (Figure 5.3).

### Integrating the Emotions Stones in Life Outside of Dramatherapy

The established practice at Roundabout is to hold in mind and integrate the systems of both school and home in order to support the wellbeing of children attending dramatherapy. A consideration of influences outside of the sessions was key to the intervention.

The interviews between the lead researcher and parents/carers and teachers provided an opportunity to hear about the impact of the children's engagement in the research at home and school and provided a rich source of data. In both schools, parents/carers turned up to every scheduled interview: strong indication of parents and carers being invested in the process and feeling heard and validated.

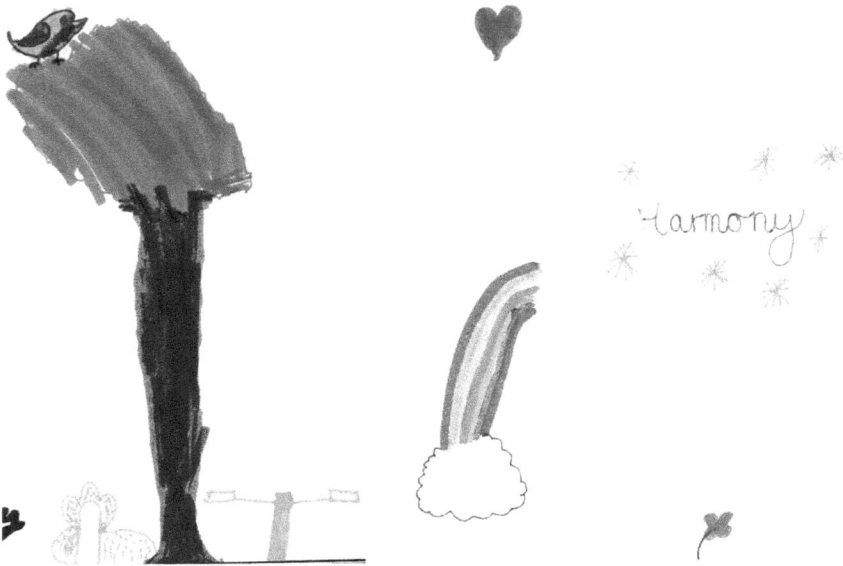

*Figure 5.3* Artwork by participants Jowey and Ginger Kitten

Parents/carers highlighted that the Emotion Stones had value and meaning outside of the dramatherapy sessions. Families reported that children were finding new ways to express themselves and their feelings at home, reducing anxiety for children as well as families. They reported an increase in their understanding that children might, for example, appear to be angry but this expression might come from a place of worry or sadness or confusion, as demonstrated by the words chosen by the children for the Emotion Stones. Adults reported that children began to be able to develop a wider emotional language to express a broader range of feelings, which in some cases highlighted additional needs and difficulties and led to identifying strategies to help support children outside of the dramatherapy. This included support in the classroom with emotional literacy and developing self-regulation techniques. Adults recognised the importance of the children being better able to identify and share what was going on for them.

Quantitative results from engagement in the parent and child anxiety-specific outcome measure (ASC/ASD, Rodgers et al., 2016) show decreased levels of anxiety in three of the four domains (performance anxiety, anxious arousal, separation anxiety, uncertainty). A qualitative analysis suggests interesting areas for further exploration between participants' perceived anxiety versus that of their parents/carers. Being aware of similarities and differences between children's and adults' results opens up new communication potentials between children and adults. In some cases, levels of anxiety had increased; but parents reported that this was because they had a better understanding of their children's levels of anxiety, due to the child's increased emotional expression as a result of attending group dramatherapy. Having better information made parents feel more equipped to support their children.

## Follow-up Interviews

Three months after the end of the intervention, the research lead met with the children and parents/carers to complete outcome measures. During these interviews, feedback about ongoing engagement with the Emotion Stones was given. For example, participant Binery's family had bought a set of stones and she had used them with her younger brother.

When invited to give feedback about being in dramatherapy, each child's comments showed a personal investment in the process of being in the group and working with the Emotion Stones. There was a sadness named and expressed by most that the group had ended, and naming of the enjoyment of being in the group and of having a consistent space to express themselves and have their voices heard, as evidenced below:

> "It's like a lot of drama and everything. It's so much fun. It's like a type of act – I'm acting out things and it makes you feel happy. You can show emotions". Mystic Justice, 10 years
> "Fun! You can talk stuff out". Binery, 9 years
> "Dramatherapy is like fun and you get to dress up, act, narrate and draw at the end … . Dramatherapy can help you calm down". Groot, 9 years

## Discussion

As outlined earlier, SaLoA's design draws on an understanding of key concerns for autistic people in relation to the prevalence and intensity of anxiety which can compromise the development of social relationships, impinge on the understanding of affect and expression of emotions, and inhibit access to educational learning (Simonoff et al., 2008; Vasa and Mazurek, 2015; Murin et al., 2016).

The study's design anticipated that children with autism coming to dramatherapy would be anxious, not necessarily about coming to dramatherapy itself, but perhaps about being in school and managing the school day or other factors in their lives. Many children with autism struggle with transitions, changes in routines, sensory processing and the intolerance of uncertainty (Boulter et al., 2014). A significant factor in the design of the study, to address and acknowledge these potential issues for group members, was the repeated session structure. Davidson (2017, p. 27),

writing about her work with autistic children, reflects that "The containment and ritual with the session structure creates a secure environment in
which the client can begin to explore and make connections".

The level of flexibility within the session structure, made possible by the
'or something else' principle (referred to earlier), invited the children to
practice managing change and unpredictability, as well as respecting
and accepting what each group member wanted to bring. Equally, the
closed group membership and longevity of the intervention (20 sessions)
enabled familiarity and predictability promoting self-regulation, sensory
balance and increased confidence for participants to be themselves and to
share the things that were important to them.

O'Nions et al. (2018) explore through a meta-synthesis study a number
of approaches taken by parents to respond to their autistic children's
presenting behaviours, including anxiety. They list nine strategies, with
third on the list being "providing structure, routine and occupation". The
importance and impact of the structure of the dramatherapy sessions were
commented on by parents and children in their evaluation of the research
project, with references to it helping children to feel more confident and
more regulated.

The environment in which the sessions took place, with a focus on the link
between sensory sensitivity and anxiety (Green and Ben-Sasson, 2010), was
also a special consideration with attention given to children's sensory experiences such as noise levels, choices of dressing up materials, and the types
of resources forming the dramatherapy kitbag.

The group process with children working together, facilitated by two
dramatherapists, led to opportunities for co-creation, group reflection and
meaning-making. Ramsden (2017, p. 61) highlights that "being alongside"
enables autistic children to develop their "capacity to tolerate others" and to
"make choices". The Emotion Stones were central to the internalising of this
process and the transfer of skills into the children's wider lives at home and
school, "Since coming to dramatherapy (child A) has seemed a lot happier in
class and is much more confident with their peers (Teacher)". Davidson
(2017, p. 27) suggests that the engagement in "embodied" experiences in
dramatherapy leads to "better integration into the day-to-day lives of this
client group".

## Conclusion

This chapter describes the innovation of integrating the Emotion Stones into the
group dramatherapy session structure and considers how this was a successful
part of the study. If this study were repeated on a larger scale, little would be
changed in the design, taking into account children's meaningful and agentic
engagement in the use of the Emotion Stones as discussed above. Individual
voice and the expression of language in response to the opportunities offered

through the session structure are congruent with findings of previous dramatherapy work (Haythorne and Seymour, 2017, p. 9; Chasen, 2011, p. 262).

A limitation of the study is the small sample. Consequently, generalisation is not possible. This could, of course, be rectified by a larger iteration. Another limitation is the precedence of recruiting only experienced dramatherapy practitioners to deliver the intervention rather than practitioners of varying levels of experience. For a replicated manualised process there would be a high likelihood of recruiting practitioners with varying levels of experience.

By describing the use of the Emotion Stones in our feasibility study, SaLoA, we intended to show how dramatherapy can provide opportunities to develop insight and emotional literacy through the expression of voice both in the group, in school and within the home environment for autistic children and children with autistic traits who are experiencing anxiety.

## Acknowledgements

A collaborative approach to the design and delivery of SaLoA is reflected in the writing of this chapter. The authorship is made up of the dramatherapists who conducted the fieldwork, the charity's chief executive officers (CEOs) – who double up as one of the facilitators and one of the clinical supervisors, and the research lead for the project. In addition, Susan Crockford (Senior Manager & Dramatherapist) provided clinical supervision, and Emma Godfrey (Senior Lecturer in Health Psychology, Kings College London) offered voluntary consultation input into the design and fieldwork stages of the study. The authors wish to thank the children, parents/carers and teachers who participated in SaLoA, and the head-teachers of the schools who agreed to host this feasibility study.

## References

Attwood, T. (2004) *Exploring feelings: Cognitive behaviour therapy to manage anxiety*. USA: Future Horizons.
Benbow, A. (2017) 'Being men: Men, Asperger's and dramatherapy', in D. Haythorne and A. Seymour (eds.) *Dramatherapy and autism*. UK: Routledge.
Boulter, C., Freeston, M., South, M. and Rodgers, J. (2014) 'Intolerance of uncertainty as a framework for understanding anxiety in children and adolescents with autism spectrum disorders', *Journal of Autism Development Disorders*, 44, pp. 1391–1402.
Braun, V. and Clarke, V. (2006) 'Using thematic analysis in psychology', *Qualitative Research in Psychology*, 3(2), pp. 77–101.

Chasen, L.R. (2011) *Social skills, emotional growth and drama therapy – Inspiring connection on the autism spectrum*. USA: Jessica Kingsley.

Davidson, R. (2017) 'Entering colourland: Working with metaphor with high-functioning autistic children', in D. Haythorne and A. Seymour (eds.) *Dramatherapy and autism*. UK: Routledge.

Dix, A. (2017) 'Becoming visible: Identifying and empowering girls on the autistic spectrum through dramatherapy', in D. Haythorne and A. Seymour (eds.) *Dramatherapy and autism*. UK: Routledge.

Dyer, N. (2017) 'Behold the tree: An exploration of the social integration of boys on the autistic spectrum in a mainstream primary school through a dramatherapy intervention', *The Journal of the British Association of Dramatherapists*, 38(2–3), pp. 80–93.

Fonagy, P. and Allison, E. (2014) 'The role of mentalizing and epistemic trust in the therapeutic relationship', *Psychotherapy*, 51(3), pp. 372–380.

Godfrey, E. and Haythorne, D. (2013) 'Benefits of dramatherapy for autism spectrum disorder: A qualitative analysis of feedback from parents and teachers of clients attending Roundabout dramatherapy sessions in schools', *Dramatherapy: The Journal of the British Association of Dramatherapists*, 35(1), pp. 20–29.

Godfrey, E. and Haythorne, D. (2017) 'An exploration of the impact of dramatherapy on the whole system supporting children and young people on the autistic spectrum', in D. Haythorne and A. Seymour (eds.) *Dramatherapy and autism*. UK: Routledge.

Green, S.A. and Ben-Sasson, A. (2010) 'Anxiety disorders and sensory over-responsivity in children with autism spectrum disorders: Is there a causal relationship?', *Journal of Autism Development Disorders*, 40, pp. 1495–1504.

Haythorne, D. (2012) 'The charity roundabout: One model of providing dramatherapy in schools', In L. Leigh, I. Gersch, A. Dix and D. Haythorne (eds.) *Dramatherapy with children, young people and schools: Enabling creativity, sociability, communication and learning*. London: Routledge.

Haythorne, D. and Seymour, A. (eds.) (2017) *Dramatherapy and autism*. UK: Routledge.

Jennings, S. (1978) *Remedial drama*. GB: A & C Black.

Jennings, S. (1993) *Playtherapy with children: A practitioner's guide*. UK: Blackwell.

Jones, P. (1996) *Drama as therapy – Theatre as living*. London: Routledge.

Jones, P., Cedar, L., Coleman, A., Haythorne, D., Mercieca, D. and Ramsden, E. (2021) *Child agency and voice in therapy*. London: Routledge.

Kerns, C.M., Kendall, P.C., Berry, L., Souders, M.C., Franklin, M.E., Schultz, R.T., Miller, J. and Herrington, J. (2014) 'Traditional and atypical presentations of anxiety in youth with autism spectrum disorder', *Journal of Autism and Developmental Disorders*, 44(1), pp. 2851–2861.

Lindkvist, M.R. (1997) *Bring white beads when you call on the healer*. UK: Garnet Miller Ltd.

Murin, M., Hellriegel, J. and Mandy, W. (2016) 'Autism spectrum disorder and the transition into secondary school: A handbook for implementing strategies in the mainstream school setting', GB: Jessica Kingsley.

Middletown Centre for Autism. (2020) *Autism and managing anxiety: Practical strategies for working with children*. USA: Routledge.

Nadeau, J., Sulkowski, M.L., Ung, D., Wood, J.J., Lewin, A.B., Murphy, T.K., Ehrenreich May, J. and Storch, E.A. (2011) 'Treatment of comorbid anxiety and autism spectrum disorders', *Neuropsychiatry*, Dec 1, (6), pp. 567–578.

O'Nions, E., Happé, F., Evers, K., Boonen, H. and Noens, I. (2018) 'How do parents manage irritability, challenging behaviour, non-compliance and anxiety in children with autism spectrum disorders? A meta-synthesis', *Journal of Autism Development Disorders*, 48, pp. 1272–1286.

Ramsden, E. (2017) 'Supporting agency, choice making and the expression of 'voice' with Kate: Dramatherapy in a mainstream primary school setting with a 9-year-old girl diagnosed with ASD and ADHAD', in D. Haythorne and A. Seymour (eds.) *Dramatherapy and Autism*, UK: Routledge.

Ramsden, E. and Jones, P. (2011) 'Ethics, children, education and therapy: Vulnerable or empowered', in A. Campbell and P. Broadhead (eds.) *Working with children and young people: Ethical debates and practices across disciplines and continents*. Germany: Peter Lang.

Ramsden, E. and Haythorne. D. (2021) 'Case study 4: Dramatherapists reducing anxiety in children with autism', in *Allied Health Professionals, transforming health, care and wellbeing for autistic people and people with a learning disability*. https://www.ahpnw.nhs.uk/media/1169/ld_autism_case_study_collection_finalv3.pdf [Accessed 30 December 2022].

Rodgers, J., Wigham, S., McConachie, H., Freeston, M., Honey, E. and Parr, J.R. (2016) 'Development of the anxiety scale for children with autism spectrum disorder (ASC-ASD)', *Autism Research*, 9, pp. 1205–1215.

Roundabout Dramatherapy (2022) Available at: http://www.roundaboutdramatherapy.org.uk [Accessed 22 March 2022].

Simonoff, E., Pickles, A., Charman, T., Chandler, S., Loucas, T. and Baird, G. (2008). 'Psychiatric disorders in children with autism spectrum disorders: Prevalence, comorbidity, and associated factors in a population-derived sample', *Journal of the American Academy of Child and Adolescent Psychiatry*, 47(8), pp. 921–929.

Van Steensel, F.J., Bogels, S.M. and Perrin, S. (2011) 'Anxiety disorders in children and adolescents with autistic spectrum disorders: A meta-analysis', *Clinical Child and Family Psychology Review*, 14(3), pp. 302–317.

Vasa, R.A. and Mazurek, M.O. (2015) 'An update of anxiety in youth with autism spectrum disorders', *Current Opinions in Psychiatry*, March, 28(2), pp. 83–90.

Yellow-door.net (2021) 'The Emotion Stones'. Available at: https://www.yellow-door.net/products/emotion-stones/ [Accessed 22 March 2022].

# Chapter 6

# Music Therapy and Children with Autism Spectrum Disorder

## A New Assessment Scale Evaluating Resilience-Informed Relationship Quality

*Laura Blauth*

## Introduction

In recent years, there has been increased awareness that symptom reduction might not be an appropriate intervention aim when working with children with autism spectrum disorder (ASD), as this approach has not reliably improved long-term outcomes and the wellbeing of affected children and their families (Straus, 2014; Silberman, 2015). Instead, strengthening protective factors and thereby fostering resilience in children with ASD has been recognised as a promising treatment model (Szatmari, 2018; Williams et al., 2018). To find out whether music therapy is a suitable intervention to enhance resilience in young children with ASD, I conducted a doctoral research study (Blauth, 2019). Using a mixed methods design, I retrospectively analysed data which had been collected but not analysed within the international randomised controlled trial of improvisational music therapy's effectiveness for children with autism (TIME-A) (Bieleninik et al., 2017). Findings from the quantitative and qualitative analyses suggest that music therapy sessions increase behaviours indicative of resilience in this client group (Blauth, 2017; Blauth and Oldfield, 2022).

In this chapter, I focus on one aspect of my research study that is of particular importance concerning resilience in children with ASD: the quality of the child-therapist relationship. A positive relationship with a supportive adult has been shown to be the primary protective factor for developing resilience (Masten, Best, and Garmezy, 1990; Luthar, 2006). This factor is especially relevant for children with ASD (Brooks and Goldstein, 2012). To investigate whether music therapy could provide autistic children with the experience of a resilience-enhancing relationship, I designed an assessment tool that measures the quality of the therapeutic relationship. In this chapter, I present the development of the tool, its application to music therapy videos, and the findings from this first study. A case study illustrates how characteristics of the clinical work relate to the quality of the child-therapist relationship and resilience.

DOI: 10.4324/9781003201656-8

### Resilience-Informed Relationship in Children with ASD

Psychological resilience refers to positive outcomes and adaptive processes in people who experience adversity (Masten and Obradović, 2006). Children are considered resilient if they do better than expected despite being exposed to risk factors, such as traumatic life events, poverty or disabilities. Protective factors, including the ability to express and regulate emotions, to deal with stress, to feel confident, and to interact comfortably with others, can moderate or mitigate these risk factors (Reivich and Shatte, 2002; Naglieri, LeBuffe and Shapiro, 2013). Longitudinal studies on resilience have shown that a positive relationship with a pro-social adult is the most significant protective factor for children at risk (Masten et al., 1990; Luthar, 2006).

Problems with social communication and interaction, as manifested by difficulties in developing, maintaining, and understanding relationships is one of the core symptoms of ASD (American Psychiatric Association, 2013). Thus, the neurodevelopmental condition must be considered a severe risk factor for the wellbeing and mental health of affected children. Unfortunately, this notion is confirmed by the high prevalence of associated psychiatric disorders. Around 70% of children with ASD have at least one other diagnosed mental-health problem, including anxiety disorders, attention deficit hyperactivity disorder, and obsessive compulsive disorder (Simonoff et al., 2008). Similarly, people with ASD are four times more likely to suffer from depression compared to their typically developing peers (Hudson, Hall and Harkness, 2018). Clinicians and researchers increasingly stress that we need to focus on strengthening protective factors of children with ASD to foster their resilience and improve long-term outcomes (Bekhet, Johnson and Zauszniewski, 2012; Kaboski, McDonnell and Valentino, 2017). Especially for this client group, the importance of positive relationships as a protective factor cannot be overestimated (Brooks and Goldstein, 2012). In a TIME-A spin-off study (Mössler et al., 2017), linear mixed-effect models confirmed that there were significant interaction effects between the quality of the therapeutic relationship and improvement in social, communication, and language skills, indicating that a positive relationship might be key for development.

To investigate this further and explore whether music therapy could provide autistic children with the experience of a positive and resilience-enhancing relationship, I conducted a video analysis using, amongst other methods, a tool assessing the child-therapist relationship with reference to the behaviour of the child.

### Review of Existing Assessment Scales

A literature search disclosed three available assessment tools that focus on measuring the therapist-client relationship and are applicable to this client group. These are the Assessment of the Quality of Relationship (AQR) (Schumacher and Calvet, 2007), the Nordoff-Robbins-Scale I: Child-Therapist

Relationship in Coactive Musical Experience (Nordoff and Robbins, 1977), and the Music Therapy Session Assessment Scale (MT-SAS) (Raglio et al., 2017). The AQR aims to assess and comprehensively classify the quality of interpersonal relationships. Four different scales with seven or eight levels each focus on the instrumental quality of the relationship, the vocal-pre-speech quality of the relationship, the physical-emotional quality of the relationship, and the therapeutic quality of the relationship. The AQR is a microanalysis method that requires extensive training. The Nordoff-Robbins-Scale I is a similarly elaborate measurement tool. It distinguishes seven levels of participation and seven levels of resistance and provides detailed rating criteria for each level. Like the AQR, the Nordoff-Robbins-Scale I is linked to a rather specific clinical approach that differed from the approach used in this study. As the analysis of the therapeutic relationship was only one aspect of a larger mixed-methods research project, both scales proved to be too extensive for the purpose of this study. More importantly, I was interested in a scale that is quick and easy to use in daily clinical practice.

The structure of the MT-SAS matches this need well. Seven behaviours in the domains of countenance, nonverbal communication, and sound-music communication are rated as predominantly absent or predominantly present, which results in a total score that conveys an overall impression of the relationship. However, as mentioned above, the analysis of the child-therapist relationship was one aspect of a larger study, which also investigated occurrences of resilience-indicating behaviours in children using time-sampling video analysis (Blauth and Oldfield, 2022). For the time-sampling analysis, videos were annotated using a coding manual. While the coding manual focused on some aspects of the child-therapist relationship, measured by codes such as 'Look' or 'Respond', it did not seem to pick up the overall quality of the relationship satisfactorily. The seven items of the MT-SAS had many overlaps with the items of the coding manual and thus the scale was not going to provide me with the additional information about the child-therapist relationship I was interested in.

## Study Approach

### Participants and Clinical Approach

For this analysis, video recordings of music therapy sessions were used that had been conducted within the international research study TIME-A at one of the sites in the UK. Children had a diagnosis of ASD and were aged between four and six years at the beginning of the intervention. Children were randomly allocated to receive individual music therapy once a week or three times a week over a period of five months. Sessions lasted approximately 30 minutes each. In the analysis of the child-therapist relationship, video recordings of sessions with 13 children were included. Of these 13 children, 6 had been randomised to the low-intensity treatment and 7 to the high-intensity treatment. Seven children were verbal while six children did not use verbal language at the beginning of treatment. In this cohort, ten children were male. Three children attended a mainstream primary school, two children a special school for children with moderate to severe learning difficulties, and eight children a special school for pupils with a diagnosis of ASD.

All three schools provided a separate room that could be used consistently for sessions. As the therapist, I made sure that a variety of appealing instruments were available. Most of the music played in sessions was live and improvised. Apart from free musical exchanges, recurring elements such as a hello and a goodbye song, familiar songs, musical games as well as movement and dance activities were incorporated into the sessions. I strive to provide an intervention that helps children to cope with their condition and become more resilient. As positive relationships have been shown to be the key factor for building resilience in children with ASD, I understand the relationship between child and therapist to be of paramount importance for any successful intervention. I try to establish trust and a positive relationship through presenting as an attentive and supportive person with a warm and welcoming attitude toward the child. Musical interactions have many similarities with early parent-infant communication, including the use of rhythm, melody, dynamics, intensity, structure, and timing as main elements of intersubjective exchange (Stern, 1985; Malloch and Trevarthen, 2009), making music an especially well-suited means to experience interpersonal relating and emotional connection. Building a positive relationship also includes providing a secure environment through, for example, maintaining the same time and room for therapy sessions, showing consistency and reliability in behaviour and responses, establishing boundaries, and preparing for interruptions and endings. Music offers the therapist the possibility to provide a secure base beyond the external environment through using musical techniques such as holding and rhythmic grounding. Music can also be used to regulate the level of excitement and arousal, to structure the session with reassuring musical activities and to provide clear beginnings and endings to each improvisation.

### Development of a New Assessment Scale

After the review of the existing scales, I decided to design a new bespoke assessment tool, which I call Assessment of Child-Therapist Relationship (ACTR). The ACTR can be completed by clinicians and researchers after a music therapy session but it is recommendable to use video recordings. Full sessions as well as shorter excerpts of sessions can be evaluated with this scale. The ACTR provides five ranks that describe the quality of relationship as 1 = difficult, 2 = slightly difficult, 3 = moderate, 4 = positive, 5 = very positive. Each of the five levels is defined by descriptions about (a) the child's emotional state and way of being in the room, (b) the child's ability to engage in reciprocal musical interactions, and (c) the child's ways of relating to the therapist. The assessment manual is shown in Figure 6.1.

## Assessment of Child-Therapist Relationship (ACTR)

| 5 = very positive | (a) Child feels secure and confident.<br>(b) Child is able to be both responsive to the therapist and in charge of the interaction. Child is able to be creative, to use humour, to share emotions and to swap roles with therapist.<br>(c) Child seems to enjoy interacting with therapist and initiates communication. The relationship is characterised by mutuality and a sense of partnership. |
| --- | --- |
| 4 = positive | (a) Child appears relaxed and comfortable, shows no signs of distress.<br>(b) Child is actively involved in music making. Child engages in turn-taking activities and responds to most prompts and musical suggestions.<br>(c) Child seems interested in interacting with therapist. |
| 3 = moderate | (a) Child appears mainly relaxed and comfortable, generally at ease in therapy situation.<br>(b) Child participates in musical activities and responds to some prompts or musical suggestions. Child may only be attentive for short periods of time so that meaningful interactions only occur occasionally.<br>(c) Child tolerates therapist and seems somewhat interested in interacting with therapist. |
| 2 = slightly difficult | (a) Child seems uncertain, wary and uneasy. When approached too directly by therapist child might become anxious, distressed or withdrawn.<br>(b) Child responds reluctantly or with resistance to musical invitations. Child's involvement in interaction can be evoked by interesting or matching music but is intermittent and fleeting.<br>(c) Child might accept therapist when interaction is on child's terms but is mainly unresponsive to therapist |
| 1 = difficult | (a) Child appears anxious, distressed or withdrawn.<br>(b) Child's engagement in musical interactions is prevented by being cut-off or isolated, or by reactions of panic, rage or rejection (such as pushing or throwing instruments).<br>(c) Child seems to be completely oblivious of therapist or child tries to actively block out and reject therapist by screaming, kicking, hitting or turning away. |

(a) Child's emotional state and way of being in the room
(b) Child's ability to engage in reciprocal musical interactions
(c) Child's way of relating to the therapist

Figure 6.1 ACTR manual

### Inter-Rater Reliability

In this study, I rated each video excerpt with one ACTR level. The excerpt selection followed a defined and tested procedure (Blauth and Oldfield, 2022). I calculated the mean level for each session, which allowed me to look at the development of the relationship mean scores for each child over the course of the therapy. Before I carried out the ACTR on all excerpts, inter-rater reliability was checked. The test was conducted on four sessions of five excerpts each, resulting in 20 excerpts. Two sessions each had been selected from two different children. For both children, one session was randomly picked from the first five, and one session from the last five therapy sessions of the child's intervention because I speculated that this would result in a broader spectrum of the observed quality of relationship. The music therapist who carried out the second rating was blinded to the phase of the treatment period. We obtained an exact agreement in 12 out of 20 excerpts. In all the remaining eight excerpts, our ratings differed by only one point (e.g., rater A and B chose 4 = positive and 5 = very positive, respectively). As the data are measured on a continuous scale, inter-rater reliability was assessed using intraclass correlation (ICC). To determine whether the two raters provided scores that were similar in absolute value, a two-way random-effects, absolute-agreement, single-measures ICC was chosen. The ICC estimate was 0.87 with a 95% confidence interval of 0.70–0.95, indicating good to excellent reliability (Koo and Li, 2016).

### Analysis

Music therapy session videos of 13 children were included in the analysis. To be able to draw statistically supported conclusions about the impact of music therapy on the development of the child-therapist relationship, the data were analysed using generalised linear mixed models (GLMM). A GLMM enables us to combine continuous and categorical predictor variables into one analysis. I was interested in the effects of the continuous, quantitative predictor variable 'session number' (i.e., intervention week) as well as in the potential effects of the categorical predictor variables 'therapy intensity' and 'verbal ability'. The model further provides the possibility to model non-linear effects. To account for differences between children and their response to therapy, I included child-ID as a random effect, consisting of random intercept and random slope. Further details about the statistical model have been published (Blauth and Oldfield, 2022). The following model was implemented:

*ACTR score ~ session number + session number$^2$ + therapy intensity + verbal ability + (1 + session number + session number$^2$ | child-ID).*

## Findings

The full-null model comparison was significant for the variable 'ACTR score' ($P < 0.001$). Values for the $P$ value, estimate, standard error, and the lower and upper confidence limits are presented for all three predictor variables in Table 6.1.

The model results are visualised in the following scatter plot, displaying the week of intervention (1–20) on the x-axis and the response value 'ACTR score' on the y-axis. Several observations conglomerating on the same point in the coordinates are represented by proportionally larger dots (Figure 6.2).

Table 6.1 Model results – relationship rating

| Predictor variable | P-value | Estimate | SE | CL lower[a] | CL upper[a] |
|---|---|---|---|---|---|
| Session number | < 0.001*** | 0.841 | 0.084 | 0.677 | 1.005 |
| Therapy intensity | 0.423 | 0.239 | 0.295 | −0.338 | 0.817 |
| Verbal ability | 0.048* | 0.630 | 0.294 | 0.053 | 1.207 |

Abbreviations: CL, Confidence limits; SE, Standard error
*$p < 0.05$. **$p < 0.01$. ***$p < 0.001$.
[a]95% confidence limits.

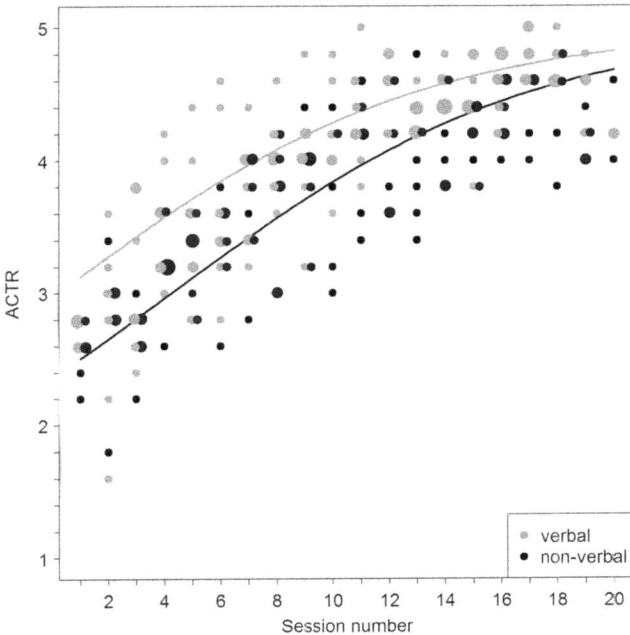

Figure 6.2 Results for 'ACTR score'

This scatter plot presents the results of the relationship rating across all 13 children. The effect of the predictor 'session number' on the ACTR score was significant ($P < 0.001$). The correlation between session number and the response was positive, which means that the relationship improved as sessions progressed. This correlation is illustrated by the upward slope of the trendlines. 'Therapy intensity' had no significant effect on the quality of the child-therapist relationship as measured by the ACTR, but the predictor 'verbal ability' was significant ($p = 0.048$). On average, verbal children, who are represented by the dots and trendline in red, received a higher score on the ACTR throughout the course of the intervention compared to the group of nonverbal children, who are represented by the dots and trendline in grey. However, it is noticeable that the two trendlines converge as the sessions progress, indicating that the ACTR scores of verbal and nonverbal children gradually became more similar.

## Case Vignette

The following case vignette will bring to life the development of one child during the study and show how our relationship evolved. For confidentiality reasons, the name of the child has been changed.

Isaac had just turned five years old when I started seeing him for music therapy. He had been assigned to the high-intensity treatment group and was offered individual music therapy sessions three times a week. Isaac attended 46 sessions over a period of 17 weeks. In his mainstream primary school, he was supported by a teaching assistant (TA) who provided one-to-one assistance and who accompanied him to the music therapy sessions. Isaac was assessed as having mild learning difficulties. In school, he paced around the classroom while performing repetitive hand movements and seemed very isolated. His teachers and parents were worried about Isaac's emotional wellbeing and his difficulties with building positive relationships with adults or children.

In the first four music therapy sessions, Isaac was constantly moving from one end of the room to the other. He picked up instruments only to discard them seconds later. The first connection with Isaac was established when I joined him in his walking, emphasising each step with a vocal sound. When he noticed that I copied his movements, he stopped for a few seconds and looked at me with a surprised expression. This moment of contact was created again when I mirrored and matched his pacing and his mood on the piano, incorporating the rhythm of his steps and the sounds he made. In this way, Isaac's expressions were reflected back to him, which might have helped him to listen and to feel listened to. My imitative responses aimed to reinforce his sense of identity and self-awareness. Isaac increasingly varied his vocal, facial and bodily expressions, and smiled and looked at me when I followed him. After these initial moments of contact, Isaac quickly became more interested in interacting with me. A striking exemplification of Isaac's

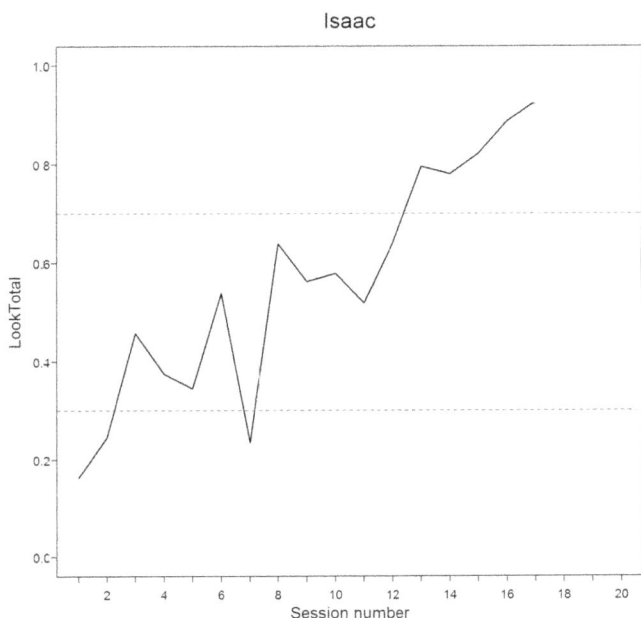

*Figure 6.3* Isaac – Proportion of looking

changing presentation is the amount of time he spent looking at me or his TA during a session. The following graph, displaying data from the time-sampling video analysis that was performed in the doctoral research study, demonstrates how this behaviour changed over the course of the intervention (Figure 6.3).

As I matched and mirrored Isaac's expressions, he experienced being in control of our music in a positive way. These empowering experiences allowed him also to respond to me and to follow my music or verbal requests at times (Figure 6.4).

Isaac's increased awareness of and responsiveness to other people around him generalised to other settings and was recognised by his parents and teachers. This change was very important for his further development. Isaac's mother commented after two months:

> I was surprised, two days ago I ask him going to bed, 'Tomorrow is music, you gonna see Miss Laura. What instruments do you use?', and he told me all the instruments. He say piano, bells, drums, even some where I don't know the name. Before he wouldn't respond.

When Isaac started his music therapy sessions, he did not use words to communicate with me, and he vocalised only occasionally. Over the course

Isaac

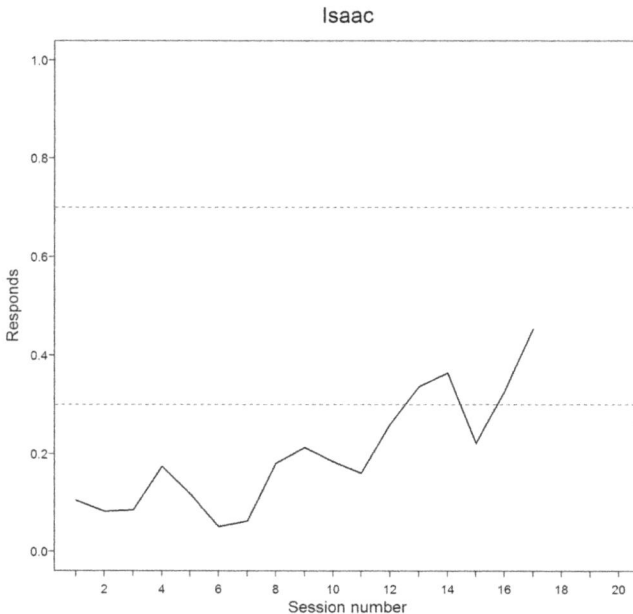

*Figure 6.4* Isaac – Proportion of responding

of therapy, he vocalised more often, possibly as a response to my almost constant singing. I tried to incorporate every vocal expression of Isaac's into my improvised music to show him that his vocalisations were heard and valued. As he was encouraged to use his voice, he started exploring it and used a wider range of sounds, pitch and volume. The high intensity of music therapy three times a week allowed for quick progress regarding Isaac's confidence and ability to use his voice (Figure 6.5).

Most encouraging was the fact, that Isaac did not only vocalise more often but also in more playful, creative and interactive ways. Similarly, his movements and his playing became more expressive. He increasingly offered his own musical ideas. The fact that Isaac had found an area in which he felt he was good at helped him to build up his self-esteem and to feel proud and happy about himself (Figure 6.6).

Isaac's mother cherished the video clips of his music therapy sessions and delighted in his enjoyment. In the following comment, she articulates how meaningful it was for her to see her son experiencing and expressing joy:

Wow, it's amazing, he is enjoying! Music helps him to communicate, to feel--, maybe to feel happy. Sometimes before he was very sad, sometimes he wasn't comfortable, but music helps him to feel happy. I'm happy because he is happy.

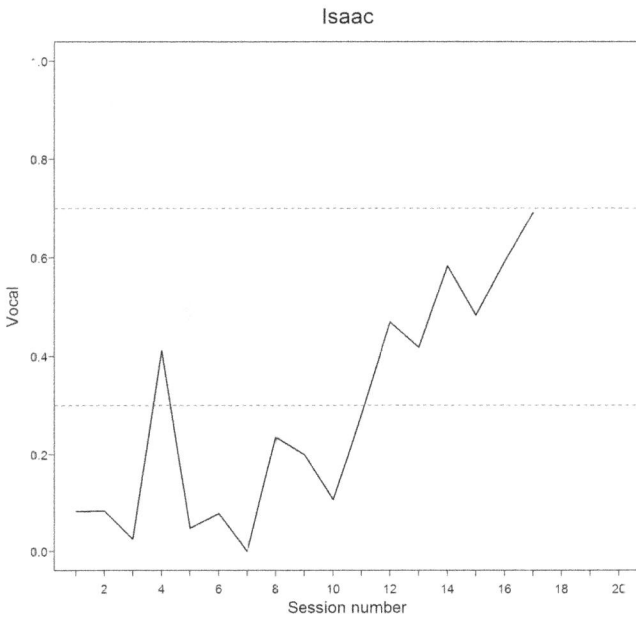

Figure 6.5 Isaac – Proportion of vocalising

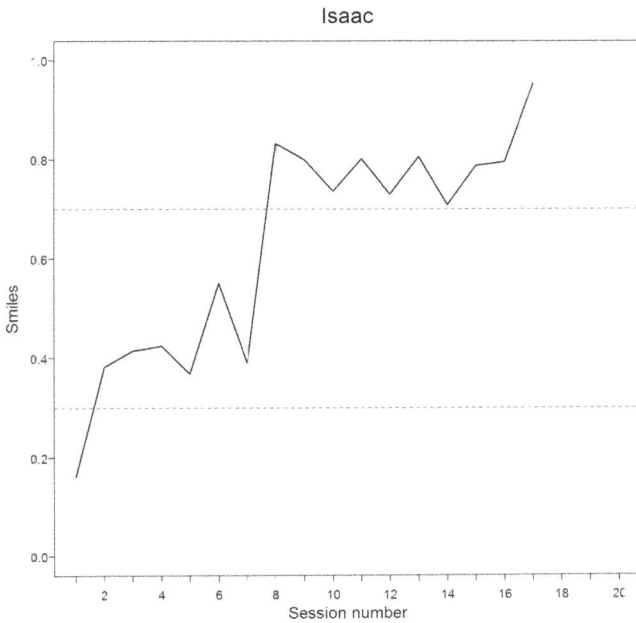

Figure 6.6 Isaac – Proportion of smiling

His mother and his teaching assistant enjoyed observing and discussing Isaac's strengths and progress, and both reported that he also started interacting and relating more with others outside the sessions. Sharing ideas with them of how to implement singing and music making at home and in his daily classroom routines further supported his positive development in different settings and contexts. For example, Isaac could use and improve his relationship skills in the music group started for him and two peers by his teaching assistant to encourage interactions with other children. As the TA had known Isaac for several months before the music therapy started and continued to work with him throughout the course of the intervention, she could give a clear account of the progress she observed:

> I can't believe how much he changed. When I think back to the first sessions and how he was a few months ago compared to now – it's like he is a different child. I mean, not a different child, but before he seemed so locked in and isolated. Maybe now we finally see what was always inside of him.

Comments from Isaac's parents and his teachers as well as my own clinical observations suggested that the strength-based music therapy approach provided Isaac with opportunities to build a positive relationship in a safe environment. To investigate this further, I applied the ACTR to his session videos. The following graph shows the development of Isaac's ACTR score over the intervention period (Figure 6.7).

In the ACTR, the child's emotional state and way of being in the room, the child's ability to engage in reciprocal musical interactions, and the child's ways of relating to the therapist are assessed. Whereas Isaac appeared uneasy and withdrawn at the beginning, he seemed comfortable and confident towards the end of the intervention. Isaac's engagement in musical interactions was intermittent and fleeting in early therapy sessions and he only responded occasionally to musical invitations. Later, he was actively involved in music making, engaged in turn-taking activities and was responsive to most musical suggestions. Furthermore, Isaac enjoyed being in charge of the musical interactions at times and he was able to be creative, to use humour and to share emotions during our mutual music making. In the first sessions, Isaac could only tolerate the therapist when the interactions were on his own terms and at times he tried to block out the therapist. Over the course of the intervention, Isaac became more interested in communicating with the therapist and even initiated interactions.

The development of Isaac's ACTR score does not only match the observations from therapist, school staff and parents but also correlates with the changes in his behaviours (looking, responding, vocalising, smiling) that were observable in the time-sampling video analysis. The music therapy

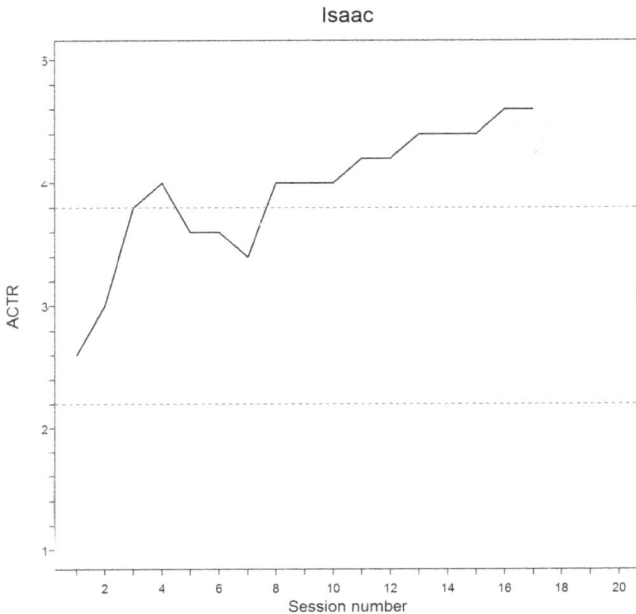

Isaac

ACTR

Session number

*Figure 6.7* Isaac – ACTR score

sessions have allowed Isaac to build a positive relationship. This experience seemed to have helped him to become also more relaxed and confident when interacting with others, and enhanced the likelihood of him becoming more resilient.

## Conclusion

Experiencing a positive relationship with an adult is a pivotal protective factor for children with ASD. It is therefore advisable to assess the relationship quality between child and therapist during an intervention in order to assess the likelihood of resilience enhancement. In this study, since none of the existing relationship measurement tools was suitable for this research and for daily clinical practice, I decided to develop a new bespoke assessment tool which I called ACTR. I applied the measurement scale ACTR to music therapy videos of 13 children with ASD. The analysis, using GLMM, showed that the quality of the child-therapist relationship improved significantly over the course of the intervention. In an inter-rater reliability test, the scale demonstrated high reliability. Furthermore, the test results correlated with the results of a time-sampling video analysis of child behaviours in the sessions. However, the measure has not undergone a strict validation procedure. The psychometric properties (i.e., validity, reliability, internal consistency) need to be tested using bigger sample sizes to make the measure accessible and useful for future music therapy research. Nevertheless, these first findings indicate that music therapy is a suitable intervention to help children with ASD experience positive relationships and develop resilience. The development of a tool like the ACTR discussed here not only captures the quality of the relationship but also contributes to focusing on resilient-informed relationships in the sessions, working on the development of children's strengths.

## References

American Psychiatric Association. (2013) *Diagnostic and statistical manual of mental disorders* (5th ed.). Arlington, VA: American Psychiatric Publishing.

Bekhet, A.K., Johnson, N.L. and Zauszniewski, J.A. (2012) 'Resilience in family members of persons with autism spectrum disorder: A review of the literature', *Issues in Mental Health Nursing*, 33(10), pp. 650–656. 10.3109/01612840.2012. 671441.

Bieleninik, Ł., Geretsegger, M., Mössler, K., Assmus, J., Thompson, G., Gattino, G., Elefant, C. et al. (2017) 'Effects of improvisational music therapy vs enhanced standard care on symptom severity among children with autism spectrum disorder: The TIME-A randomized controlled trial', *JAMA*, 318(6), pp. 525–535. 10.1001/jama.2017.9478.

Blauth, L.K. (2017) 'Improving mental health in families with autistic children: Benefits of using video feedback in parent counselling sessions offered alongside music therapy', *Health Psychology Report*, 5(2), pp. 138–150. 10.5114/hpr.2017. 63558.

Blauth, L. (2019) 'Music therapy and parent counselling to enhance resilience in young children with autism spectrum disorder: A mixed methods study', PhD diss., Anglia Ruskin University.

Blauth, L. and Oldfield, A. (2022) 'Research into increasing resilience in children with autism through music therapy: Statistical analysis of video data', *Nordic Journal of Music Therapy*. 10.1080/08098131.2022.2044893.

Brooks, R. and Goldstein, S. (2012) *Raising resilient children with autism spectrum disorders: Strategies for maximizing their strengths, coping with adversity, and developing a social mindset.* New York, NY: McGraw-Hill.

Hudson, C.C., Hall, L. and Harkness, K.L. (2018) 'Prevalence of depressive disorders in individuals with autism spectrum disorder: A meta-analysis', *Journal of Abnormal Child Psychology*, 47(1), pp. 165–175. 10.1007/s10802-018-0402-1.

Kaboski, J., McDonnell, C.G. and Valentino, K. (2017) 'Resilience and autism spectrum disorder: Applying developmental psychopathology to optimal outcome', *Review Journal of Autism and Developmental Disorder*, 4(3), pp. 175–189. 10. 1007/s40489-017-0106-4.

Koo, T.K. and Li, M.-Y. (2016) 'A guideline of selecting and reporting intraclass correlation coefficients for reliability research', *Journal of Chiropractic Medicine*, 15(2), pp. 155–163. 10.1016/j.jcm.2016.02.012.

Luthar, S.S. (2006) 'Resilience in development: A synthesis of research across five decades', in D. Cicchett and D.J. Cohen (eds.) *Developmental psychopathology: Risk, disorder, and adaptation*. Hoboken, NJ: Wiley, 739–795.

Malloch, S. and Trevarthen, C. (eds.) (2009) *Communicative musicality: Exploring the basis of human companionship*. Oxford, England: Oxford University Press.

Masten, A.S., Best, K.M. and Garmezy, N. (1990) 'Resilience and development: Contributions from the study of children who overcome adversity', *Development and Psychopathology*, 2(4), pp. 425–444. 10.1017/S0954579400005812.

Masten, A.S. and Obradović, J. (2006) 'Competence and resilience in development', *Annals of the New York Academy of Sciences: Resilience in Children*, 1094, pp. 13–27. 10.1196/annals.1376.003.

Mössler, K., Gold, C., Assmus, J., Schumacher, K., Calvet, C., Reimer, S., Iversen, G. and Schmid, W. (2017) 'The therapeutic relationship as predictor of change in music therapy with young children with autism spectrum disorder', *Journal of Autism and Developmental Disorders*, 49 (7), pp. 2795–2809. 10.1007/s10803-017-3306-y.

Naglieri, J.A., LeBuffe, P.A. and Shapiro, V.B. (2013) 'Assessment of social-emotional competencies related to resilience', in S. Goldstein and R. Brooks (eds.) *Handbook of resilience in children*. New York, NY: Springer, pp. 261–272.

Nordoff, P. and Robbins, C. (1977) *Creative music therapy: Individualized Treatment for the handicapped child*. John Day Company.

Raglio, A., Gnesi, M., Monti, M.C., Oasi, O., Gianotti, M., Attardo, L., Gontero, G. et al. (2017) 'The music therapy session assessment scale (MT-SAS): Validation of a new tool for music therapy process evaluation', *Clinical Psychology and Psychotherapy*, 24 (6), pp. O1547–O1561. 10.1002/cpp.2115.

Reivich, K. and Shatte, A. (2002) *The resilience factor: Seven essential skills for overcoming life's inevitable obstacles*. New York, NY: Broadway Books.

Schumacher, K. and Calvet, C. (2007) 'The "AQR-instrument" (assessment of the quality of relationship): An observation instrument to assess the quality of a relationship', in T. Wosch and T. Wigram (eds.) *Microanalysis in music therapy: Methods, techniques and applications for clinicians, researchers, educators and students*. London, England: Jessica Kingsley Publishers, pp. 79–91.

Silberman, S. (2015) *NeuroTribes: The legacy of autism and the future of neurodiversity*. New York, NY: Penguin Random House LLC.

Simonoff, E., Pickles, A., Charman, T., Chandler, S., Loucas, T. and Baird, G. (2008) 'Psychiatric disorders in children with autism spectrum disorders: Prevalence, comorbidity, and associated factors in a population-derived sample', *Journal of the American Academy of Child and Adolescent Psychiatry*, 47(8), pp. 921–929. 1097/ CHI.0b013e318179964f.

Stern, D.N. (1985) *The interpersonal world of the infant: A view from psychoanalysis and developmental psychology*. New York, NY: Karnac.

Straus, J. (2014) 'Music therapy and autism: A view from disability studies', *Voices: A World Forum for Music Therapy*, 14(3). 10.15845/voices.v14i3.785.

Szatmari, P. (2018) 'Risk and resilience in autism spectrum disorder: A missed translational opportunity?', *Developmental Medicine and Child Neurology*, 60(3), pp. 225–229. 10.1111/dmcn.13588.

Williams, D.L., Siegel, M., Mazefsky, C.A. and Autism and Developmental Disorders Inpatient Research Collaborative (ADDIRC). (2018) 'Problem behaviors in autism spectrum disorder: Association with verbal ability and adapting/coping skills', *Journal of Autism and Developmental Disorders*, 48(11), pp. 3668–3677. 10.1007/s10803-017-3179-0.

# Part II

# Blooming Hatchlings – Arts Therapies with Young People and Adults on the Autism Spectrum

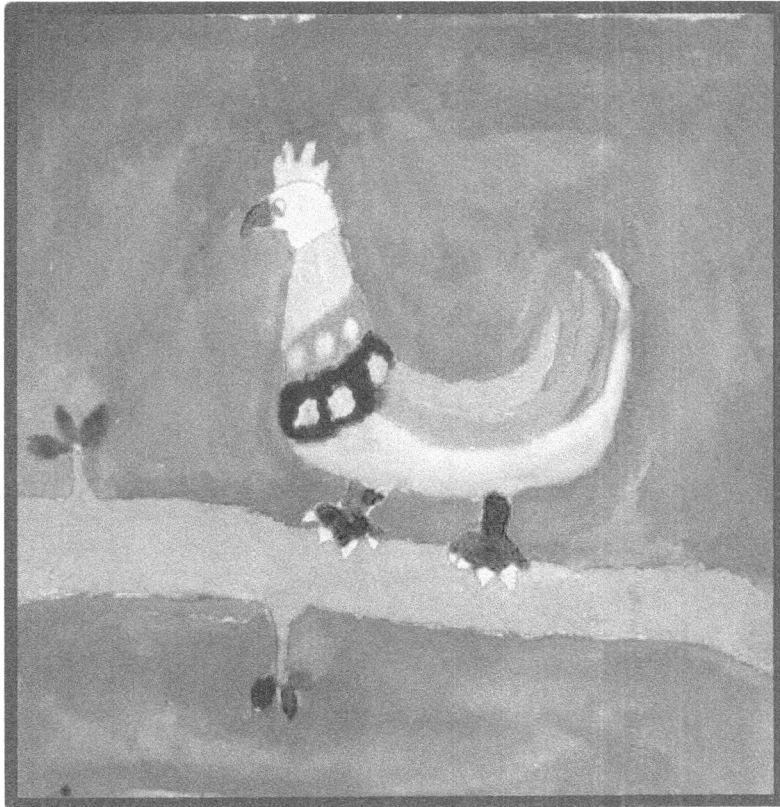

Chapter 7

# The Impact of Mirroring in Dance Movement Therapy on Empathy and Relating in Autism Spectrum Disorder

## A Secondary Reflexive Research

*Sabine C. Koch and KerryLyn Kercher*

## Introduction

Historically, mirroring in dance and music has been used in many cultures all over the globe for celebration, community strengthening, connection building and healing purposes (Schott-Billmann, 2015). In the current de-colonisation movement in the field, Dance Movement Therapy (DMT) is moving towards acknowledging its roots in non-western traditions (Nemetz, 2006; Caldwell and Leighton, 2018; Nichols, 2019). This chapter is written from the perspective of two white, cisgender, able-bodied authors, one from Germany and one from the USA, and we acknowledge the cultural and subcultural limitations this combination implies. In the following, we are providing a brief overview of the recent history of mirroring techniques in Western DMT and DMT research.

According to dance therapist Marian Chace, who introduced the technique in psychiatric hospitals, mirroring should reflect the quality as well as the shape of the movement (Sandel, Chaiklin and Lohn, 1993). The Chace approach has humanistic (Rogers, 1951), interpersonal (Sullivan, 1953), participatory and resource-oriented foundations (Sandel, 1993). The "how" of the movement (quality) can be more important than the "what" (the form or shape): Does the movement rise with softness in an airy quality, or does it lift abruptly and stop in a fixed position? Is the movement decelerating in speed? Is the emphasis on the same beat as the partner's? Thus, within the context of DMT, mirroring does not refer to a mechanical imitation, but the use of kinaesthetic empathy and attention to quality of movement through the mindful synchronisation with the other.

In bodily mirroring, the promotion of the ability to empathise takes place primarily on an implicit and nonverbal level (Fraenkel, 1983; Blair, 2005; Devereaux, 2012; Carr and Winkielman, 2014). By directly picking up and (mutually) expanding movement qualities of an individual, multiple systems of

DOI: 10.4324/9781003201656-10

the person are activated: personal attentiveness, interpersonal engagement, and environmental awareness (e.g., connection to self, connection to others, and connection to the environment). Developmental learning can thus take place on different levels, and interpersonal flexibility can be expanded. In 2010, Marianne Eberhard-Kächele introduced a detailed theory/taxonomy on developmental mirroring. Based on the research of Stern (2010), Kestenberg (1975), Schore (1994), Sodian (2005) and others, she describes nine stages of mirroring and their relation to psychopathology (Eberhard-Kächele, 2010, 2012). This framework provides the researcher and practitioner with a rich set of hypotheses and intervention approaches to work from.

If we follow Merleau-Ponty (1962), the basis of the ability to resonate lies in embodied kinaesthetics, that is, in the proprioceptive sense of the living body. Body work and DMT should therefore be particularly suitable for restoring or improving the ability for intra- and inter-bodily resonance. Interpersonal emotional resonance with others is a challenge for individuals with ASD and requires particular attention and adaptations when mirroring is used. Dance movement therapists mirror interventions in groups, and partner exercises can therefore presumably improve not only body awareness but also body image, body self-efficacy, and the ability to attune to others (Manders et al., 2021) as outlined in this chapter.

## Study Approach

We have used a secondary reflexive methodology (Sköldberg and Alvesson, 2000) as a desk method. Reflection means interpreting one's own assumptions, findings and practices by looking at one's own perspectives from those of others and by subjecting one's own assumptions to critical review (Sköldberg and Alvesson, 2000). Reflective research involves researching one's own theoretical suppositions about practices – "careful interpretation and reflection" (p. 5), in the author's words an "interpretation of interpretation" (p. 6).

The process of reflective research includes reality (re)construction and thinking about the given conditions and the way in which underlying theory, cultural values and political perspectives impact interaction (Sköldberg and Alvesson, 2000). Steps applied in the chapter were (a) a critical review of our own past studies, which resulted in a model, and (b) the critical reflection of our own and others' findings, which resulted in a new perspective on the role of sensorimotor empathy and its links to attachment.

### The Mirroring Intervention Protocol

#### Goals of the Mirroring Intervention Protocol

Our mirroring intervention protocol (MIP) was developed in 2012, when we started researching the benefits of mirroring for ASD in an evidence-based way. The objective of the MIP is to promote empathy, social competence, body awareness, and boundary awareness between self and others. Its embodied approach aims to provide an expressive training platform for the increase of emotional empathy, as well as the development of nonverbal skills in the everyday interactions of severely impaired client groups. Nonverbal communication skills refer to abilities of spatio-temporal coordination between two or more interaction partners in everyday life. The sensorimotor level is thereby assumed to have a direct impact on the emotional level (Figure 7.1). In this example, you can see how an embodied approach such as DMT can create a flow of information between a physical experience and the emotional and cognitive processes. It is believed that through the mirroring intervention, this spatio-temporal coordination between two or more interaction partners can be first experienced and then learned.

*Overview of the Mirroring Intervention Protocol*

The intervention programme "Therapeutic Mirroring for ASD" and its MIP protocol were developed by Koch in a collaboration with the Section for Phenomenological Philosophy and Psychotherapy (T. Fuchs) at Heidelberg University Hospital in the EU-project TESIS (Toward an Embodied Science of Intersubjectivity). It was tested and manualised in a feasibility study (Koch et al., 2015), and applied in a randomised controlled trial (Hildebrandt et al., 2016; Mastrominico et al., 2018). Three institutions for persons with ASD in the Rhein-Neckar region participated in the studies. The MIP intervention is taught as part of the DMT curriculum at SRH Hochschule Heidelberg.

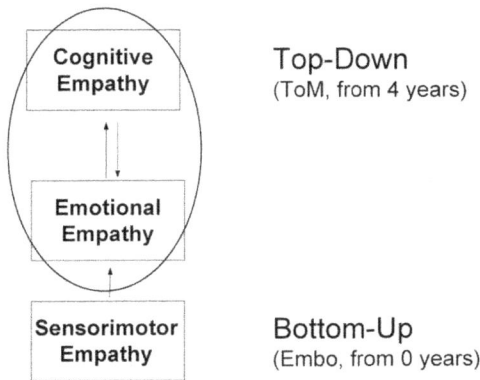

*Figure 7.1* The impact of sensorimotor empathy on emotional empathy as attained by therapeutic mirroring

The DMT intervention consists of four parts, three predominantly non-verbal and one predominantly verbal. It is offered in seven to ten sessions of one hour each by a therapist and a co-therapist, one session per week. Table 7.1 provides an overview of the intervention.

If necessary, the individual therapist used additional methods to activate resources and strengthen the participants' ability to interact and express themselves, or to structure the programme. The Embodied Intersubjectivity Scale (EIS, Fuchs and Koch, 2014) was employed to measure the success of the mirroring intervention (employed in session 2 and in the penultimate session).

### Rationale for the Mirroring Intervention Protocol: Improvements of Empathy from an Embodied Perspective

The Mirroring Intervention Protocol (MIP) aims to improve various outcomes through work on the body/movement level. Compared to the cognitive understanding of empathy as in the Theory of Mind (ToM) approaches (Baron-Cohen, Leslie and Frith, 1985; Baron-Cohen and Wheelwright, 2004) and the resulting programmes for empathy promotion (Klinger and Williams, 2009), embodiment approaches (Gallagher, 2004; Trevarthen, 2004) have a more pronounced sensorimotor understanding of empathy and describe impairments of the disorder at the intracorporeal level (Fuchs and Koch, 2014). Through this understanding, autism can be diagnosed earlier and treatment can be implemented earlier – ideally from birth onwards (the below DMT intervention is designed for individual support and has been described for children from two years on; Adler, 1970). The motoric accompaniment of the child (by moving along and mirroring) leads to (a) contingency formation, and (b) sensorimotor empathy (resonance, attunement, kinaesthetic empathy), and from there to (c) emotional empathy. This process can, but does not have to, be accompanied by cognitive empathy. Note that both theory of mind and embodiment approach aim at improving emotional empathy from two different sides, mind and body, and can therefore *complement each other*.

Mirroring and spontaneous imitation play an important role in the development of empathy, belonging, and rapport (Chartrand and van Baaren, 2009; Miles, Nind and Macrea, 2009). Nonverbal aspects of empathy were also described by Blair (2005), who speaks of "motor empathy", Tortora (2005), as well as Kestenberg's (1975; Kestenberg and Sossin, 1979) "kinaesthetic empathy" and Shai and Belsky's (2011) "parental embodied mentalising", referring to nonverbal affective intention patterns in early childhood interaction with the caregiver. Blair (2005) assumes that motor empathy is neurally anchored in functions of the mirror neuron system (Rizzolatti et al., 1996; Ramachandran and Oberman, 2006). Moreover, for empathy to emerge, exteroceptive, interoceptive and proprioceptive components of the person must be mature enough to allow integration of internal

*Table 7.1* Overview of the mirroring intervention protocol MI=

| | |
|---|---|
| **Warm-Up (approx. 10 min.):**<br><br>Mirroring in a circle: a low-threshold structured introduction, alternatively<br><br>**a.) Chace Circle**, i.e. free movement, picking up the movements of the participants by the leader, addressing them by name, naming the movement, modification of the movements (e.g. increasing, decreasing the size), or<br><br>**b.) Warm-up circle**, in which each patient in turn gives a movement in the direction of the circle, which is taken up by all, address by name, meaningful movement supplement in the sense of a completely functional warm-up by the therapist. | **Goal:** Initiation. reflection and variation in movement (safely in group/room).<br><br>**Warm-up:** Bringing participants together as a group; creating group cohesion; safe space (prerequisite for expression); everyone feels seen, valued, and supported (by picking up movements); relationship building; arrival at self and group; body awareness, functional desire, expansion of movement repertoire and sensorimotor skills. |
| **Dyadic mirroring (approx. 15 min.):**<br><br>Two partners work together. First, partner A leads in movement and partner B follows and in the second song, partner B leads and partner A follows.<br><br>Following means: mirroring oriented to the mirror axis, mirroring more the quality of the movement than the form, being respectful and mindful of the partner. Then, to the third song, "free movement" takes place, where both partners can make their own movements, but should continue to relate to each other ("stay in contact"). On the basis of this last part, an assessment is then made as to whether the participants show preferences for concordant modal mirroring (mirroring oriented to the mirror axis) or for concordant opposite mirroring (mirroring oriented to their own body axis) or how they generally develop with regard to the developmental sequence of mirroring (cf. Eberhard, 2009; 2010). | **Goal:** Emotional empathy through nonverbal sharing in the dyad.<br><br>By practicing dyadic attunement in (a) alternating roles (leading and following) and (b) shared free movement (synchronicity, differentiation, individuation, permeability, play, clash & repair), (c) empathic emotion (+ cognition) is possible; sensory-motor, interactive, emotional and affective skills as well as interaction-related attentiveness in nonverbal dialogue are trained. Furthermore, the nonverbal approach to the other person, the increasing permeability, flexibility and variability of forms of expression with simultaneous reduction of anxiety. |

*(Continued)*

Table 7.1 (Continued)

| Baum Circle (approx. 30 min.): | |
|---|---|
| This method again takes place in the group, usually in a large circle. One participant initiates the most authentic possible movements to an entire piece of music ("doing their thing"; this is initially demonstrated by the therapist as a model). The music should be chosen and brought along by the participant themselves; the criterion for the selection should be the personal (emotional) significance. The whole group follows the participant in his movements to this music, taking into account the principles of mindful mirroring ("being with the person"). Approximately four participants per session take their turn one after the other. | **Goal:** Emotional empathy through nonverbal sharing in the group.<br><br>- For initiating participants: Affect expression (to personally significant music), training of sensorimotor, emotional and communication skills.<br><br>- With co-moving participants: Bodily resonance, attunement, kinaesthetic empathy sensory-motor empathy (sensorimotor and affective skill), and finally empathic emotion (+ cognition) (emotional and affective skill). |
| **Verbal reflection (approx. 5 min. \*):** | |
| Then the group sits down and reflects on the lesson (if necessary with the help of a worksheet). First, the initiating participant X reports how it was for them to move in the Baum circle to the music (Did I express what I wanted? How was it that the others mirrored me?), then the group members tell how it was for them to move with X (What did I feel? Could I empathise? etc.). Then there is room to discuss the rest of the session. | **Goal:** Empathic emotion / cognition & insight through verbal sharing with group. Sharing of subjective experience with focus on emotions in verbal feedback (emotional and cognitive empathy), empathic reactions and regulation between participants (emotive, cognitive, sensory, motivational and social skills); boundary setting; self-perception and perception of others; perception of group and safe space; reflection and feedback. |

Source: ("Therapeutic Mirroring" Programme; Koch et al., 2015, Mastrominico et al., 2018; see also indications and contraindications for ASD, described in Koch, 2020).
Note: *The time allocation is adapted to autistic participants; for other participant groups, we recommend extending the verbal reflection to approx. 20 min, within a session of one hour.

and external perception. This is probably one of the difficulties in autism (see Mundy, Gwaltney and Henderson, 2010). DMT is therefore a promising approach for individuals with ASD (McGarry and Russo, 2011; Behrends, Mueller and Dziobek, 2012). Bodywork and body procedures can have a strengthening effect on sensory aspects of empathy. Without claiming to be a theory system, Figure 7.2 lists aspects of empathy, its nonverbal antecedents, and consequences relevant to this chapter in an overview.

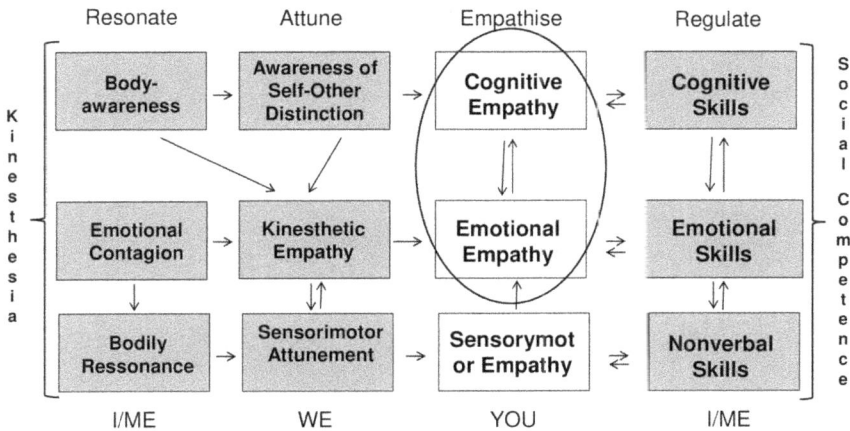

*Figure 7.2* Through the body to empathy: hypothesised relationships between empathy-related concepts at the sensorimotor, emotional and cognitive levels

As shown in Figure 7.2, kinaesthetic (Husserl, 1952) forms the basis of bodily resonance, emotional contagion (Hatfield, Cacioppo and Rapson, 1994), and body awareness. This, in turn, forms the basis for attunement to the other (interbody resonance, Fuchs, 2012; kinaesthetic empathy, Kestenberg, 1975; Fischman, 2008) which leads to different types of empathy. Empathy is regulated by skills (cognitive, emotional, and sensorimotor) that include the important functions of control and suppression (inhibition) which in turn form the basis of social competence (Reichow and Volkmar, 2010). Following this approach, social competence is decisively shaped by sensorimotor aspects. However, sensorimotor empathy is often not the subject of theories and instructions for empathy measurement and promotion. If we assume that it creates the basis of emotional and cognitive empathy in many respects, it must also be taken into account.

Other components of empathy development in terms of sensorimotor empathy include imitation (Fraenkel, 1983), echoing (a time-delayed form of imitation; Fraenkel, 1983), and adjustment (Kestenberg, 1975; Kestenberg Amighi et al., 1999). Most of these components tend to be unidirectional – in the sense of "I conform to you" – and do not describe reciprocal or symmetrical processes. However, because of this simple structure, they can provide important services for the initiation of sensorimotor attunement at the "we" level, especially when spontaneous resonance is impaired. Synchronising (Ramsayer and Tschacher, 2011), on the other hand, is based on the system level of the "we" from the very beginning, with the dyad forming a separate unit. In the programme through the MIP, one's own body

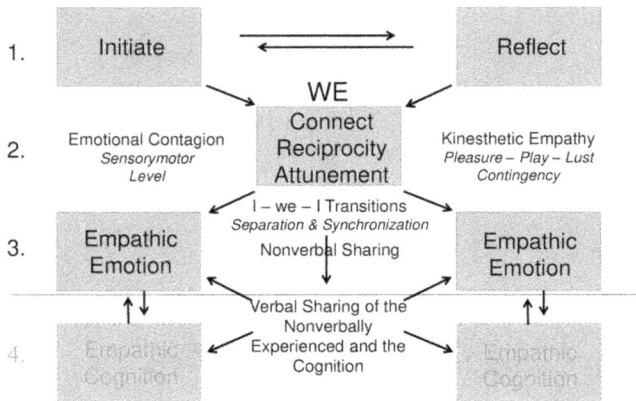

*Figure 7.3* The empathy process in the therapeutic mirroring protocol

*Note:* Three nonverbal steps and one verbal step in empathy development in the "Therapeutic Mirroring" sensorimotor training MIP (Koch et al., 2015); the verbalisation is an important therapeutic step, but not a necessary one for therapeutic change to occur.

awareness and the strengthening of the competence to differentiate between self and other is trained as the basis of kinaesthetic and emotional empathy. Only when I know that I am "I" and you are "YOU" can a real engagement and empathy develop (and a real "WE"; see Figure 7.3).

## Empirical Findings

### Effects of the Intervention

In the feasibility study, positive results were found for participants with autism (Koch et al., 2015). In a sample of N=31 participants (17 EC; 14 KG) in a rehabilitation facility in the Rhein-Neckar-Region (Germany), there was a significant improvement in body perception, social competence, boundary perception of self and others and wellbeing, following seven weekly sessions led by a dance movement therapist, a co-therapist and several student assistants. Empathy ability (Caruso and Mayer, 1998; own translation) and Saarbrücker Persönlichkeitsfragebogen - Empathic Concern (SPF-EC) as a subscale of emotional empathy (from the Interpersonal Reactivity Index (IRI), Davis, 1983; in the translation of Paulus, 2009) also improved in the intervention group, but failed to reach statistical significance. However, nonverbal empathic abilities improved, as evidenced by qualitative observations according to the mirroring taxonomy of Eberhard-Kächele (2012). At the end of the intervention, the participants of the study showed an increase in contralateral mirroring, which was further advanced into complementary mirroring (play behaviour with complementary roles, such as captor and captive; hider and seeker). Observations of this were made in "free dance" with the partner. Partners were either other participants on the autism spectrum or student assistants. An interesting observation was the unexpectedly good skills, and thus important resources, the participants all displayed in terms of mirroring. Some participants imitated their partners almost perfectly and needed the hint that it was more about "resonating with the qualities of the partner's movement" (the "how" of the movement) rather than a perfect technical imitation of the form (the "what" of the movement). The discovery of this resource in themselves immediately led participants to a self-efficacy experience ("I can" experience, Husserl, 1952), and the experience of pleasure/fun with this form of therapy. Plus, as noted by the behaviour therapist on staff, they practised a life skill that may help them to find friends or a partner, when they use it in the field.

In the randomised controlled trial (RCT) of Mastrominico and colleagues (2018) of the EU-project TESIS, we evaluated DMT for autism with the same protocol. In this study, we used the Cognitive and Emotional Empathy Questionnaire (CEEQ) (Savage et al., 2010) to measure empathy, as it includes emotional empathy - with some items at the nonverbal level (especially emotional contagion; Hatfield, Cacioppo and Rapson, 1994), and this therefore seemed to be even more suited for our methodology and target domain than the empathy scale of Caruso and Mayer (1998). In addition, the changes in empathy in movement (i.e., at the sensorimotor and whole-body levels) – operationalised according to Garcia-Perez, Lee and Hobson (2007) – were assessed by external raters using movement analysis and by the study therapists (all qualified dance movement therapists). At the end of every second hour of therapy, the extent to which the participants felt close to themselves, the group, the mirror partner and the therapist, how involved they were and how well they were able to perceive the boundaries between themselves and others were recorded. Again, results suggested that empathy as measured with the CEEQ did not significantly increase after the intervention (Mastrominico et al., 2018).

### Acceptance of the Intervention

Acceptance of the MIP protocol has been good in all contexts where it was tested. With participants on the autism spectrum, it has been particularly high, as participants quickly became aware of their resources in this area. Experience with the programme suggests that participants with severe limitations of empathy respond well to the programme and also feel that they are practicing meaningful skills or acquiring methods to make better use of their existing skills. The therapists appreciated the structuring and the simultaneous freedom that the protocol offers.

## Discussion

Critically, what makes the "mirroring" idea and related phenomena appealing is the possibility that they reveal a non-representational relation to others. (Carr and Winkielman, 2014, referring to Gallagher, 2007, Hutto, 2007, and Sinigaglia, 2009)

### Reflection on the Effects

In sum, the presented intervention programme "Therapeutic Mirroring for ASD" (DMT mirroring interventions; Koch et al., 2015; Koch et al., 2019; Mastrominico et al., 2018) shows an increase in wellbeing (particularly relaxation), body perception, boundary perception between self and other and social competency, but no strong findings regarding empathy enhancement in participants with autism from the studies.

Why did the studies of Koch et al. (2015) and the Mastrominico et al. (2018) not show a significant improvement of empathy after the DMT interventions? First, only components of cognitive and emotional empathy were measured, using the scale of Caruso and Mayer (1998) and the SPF-E emotional empathy subscale of the IRI (Davis, 1983) in the study of Koch and colleagues (2015), and the CEEQ (Savage et al., 2010) in the study of Mastrominico et al. (2018), but the instruments did not include empathy on a sensorimotor level. Qualitative observations using Eberhard-Kächele's developmental mirroring taxonomy helped to identify changes (Eberhard-Kächele, 2012).

Several other parameters changed favourably after the DMT intervention, such as wellbeing, relaxation, social competence, and self-other distinction (see Koch et al., 2015; Mastrominico et al., 2018), but not empathy. The length of the intervention and the size of the sample should also be considered here: while wellbeing can change more easily, while changes in structural features such as empathy may need longer and be more complex to change. In the search for new relational correlates co-varying with mirroring in DMT, we are now looking at Feniger-Schaal et al. (2018) who found *attachment* to be another important correlate of mirroring.

### Reflections on Attachment and Mirroring

Attachment is "the emotional bond between a human infant [...] and its parent figure or caregiver; it is developed as a step in establishing a feeling of security and demonstrated by calmness while in the parent's or caregiver's presence" (APA Dictionary of Psychology, 2021). Attachment is the relational clue between persons, our human dimension of bonding, the most influential ties to others that exist in our lives, physically, emotionally, and psychologically.

In a small group laboratory experiment, Feniger-Schaal and others (2018) found that participants who were securely attached mirrored more freely with others than participants with any other (of the four major) attachment patterns. This means Feniger-Schaal et al. identified a *behavioral correlate for attachment* in a laboratory mirroring task – a groundbreaking finding, since so far attachment styles could only be measured by self-report questionnaires or interviews. Feniger-Schaal and colleagues' (2018) findings bear much potential for research and therapeutic work, helping to build attachment from scratch, and to support the secondary gain of secure attachment from the body level.

Future questions

- Will clinical and other studies with participants with ASD find similar results to the laboratory results of Feniger-Schaal et al. (2018), or will there be important differences?
- What can we learn about mirroring as a therapeutic mechanism (see Shuper-Engelhard, 2019)?
- Since attachment is such a basic human dimension, with a crucial functional value for all mammals, what can we learn about the biological, psychological and epistemological function of mirroring?

### Reflections on the Intervention Programme

An important question is whether the sensorimotor and kinaesthetic empathy promoted by the programme promotes does in fact have an impact on emotional and cognitive empathy? Does it also have traceable consequences for the improvement of the participants' skills and social competence? Participants quickly discovered the movement level as a resource and subsequently participated in the "Therapeutic Mirroring for ASD" programme with joy and fun. Problematic for the participants with autism, however, was the verbal closing part of the therapy programme; almost none of them succeeded in verbalising the experiences and the progress made on the nonverbal level. The participants verbally seemed to be cut off from their experience, which we attributed, among other things, to the high degrees of *alexithymia* (the inability to recognise or verbalise one's own emotions; measured with the TAS-26 in the translation of Kupfer, Brosig and Brähler, 2001; which was a control variable in our studies). However, we found that participants were better able to verbally communicate aspects of their experience in the group, if they had previously read three final questions on a sheet and answered them for themselves, possibly because the threat of speaking directly about feelings in the social situation was lessened.

Interestingly, participants with autism (just as neuro-typical participants) experienced that it was nice and easy to move with some people, and difficult with others; these were different people for different participants, so that the "WE"-level always had a strong emergent component and was not predictable. Personal friendships and preferences for individual participants played a role in partner choice. While this was an unpredictable variable for the design, it is also a strength of the programme: *perceiving preferences* (those in which interactions flow easily vs do not flow) is already an important achievement for participants with autism. We were content to observe that participants all reached that point of perceiving preferences for some partners over others and that the programme seemed to strengthen the ties to the ones chosen for the mirroring task (Manders et al., 2021).

## Conclusion

In sum, our work with the present intervention programme in relation to persons with ASD, together with other recent findings, shows that working on sensorimotor and kinaesthetic aspects opens up new possibilities in diagnosis and therapy for clients; this way of working also brings challenges regarding empathy and relating. The studies failed to show a significant increase in empathy after mirroring, which may be due to the items insufficiently capturing changes on the sensorimotor level. Two other relational measures improved: self-reported social competence and boundary perception of self and others. Common measurements, which capture emotional and cognitive aspects of empathy, need to be extended to include kinaesthetic aspects of empathy and integrate the sensorimotor dimension into existing empathy research. Attachment seems to be directly related to mirroring in movement, and clinical studies are warranted to reflectively investigate this connection.

## References

Adler, J. (1970) *Looking for Me* (Video). Berkeley, CA: Berkeley Extension.

APA Dictionary of Psychology (2021) 'Attachment'. Retrieved 27 December 2021 from https://dictionary.apa.org/attachment (American Psychological Association)

Baron-Cohen, S., Leslie, A.M. and Frith, U. (1985) 'Does the autistic child have a 'theory of mind'?', *Cognition*, 21(1), pp. 37–46.

Baron-Cohen, S. and Wheelwright, S. (2004) 'The empathy quotient: An investigation of adults with Asperger syndrome or high functioning autism, and normal sex differences', *Journal of Autism and Developmental Disorders*, 34(2), pp. 163–175.

Behrends, A., Mueller, S. and Dziobek, I. (2012) 'Moving in and out of synchrony: A concept for a new intervention fostering empathy through interactional movement and dance', *The Arts in Psychotherapy*, 39, pp. 107–116.

Blair, R.J.R. (2005) 'Responding to the emotions of others: Dissociating forms of empathy through the study of typical and psychiatric populations', *Consciousness and Cognition*, 14(4), pp. 698–718.

Caldwell, C. and Leighton, L.B. (2018) *Oppression and the body: Roots, resistance, and resolutions*. Berkeley, CA: North Atlantic Books.

Carr, E.W. and Winkielman, P. (2014) 'When mirroring is both simple and "smart": How mimicry can be embodied, adaptive, and non-representational', *Frontiers in Human Neuroscience*, 8, p. 505. doi: 10.3389/frhum.2014.00505

Caruso, D.R. and Mayer, J.D. (1998) *A measure of emotional empathy for adolescents and adults*. Unpublished Manuscript.

Chartrand, T.L. and van Baaren, R. (2009) 'Human mimicry', *Advances in Experimental Social Psychology*, 41, pp. 219–274. doi:10.1016/S0065-2601(08)00405-X

Davis, M.H. (1983) 'Measuring individual differences in empathy: Evidence for a multidimensional approach', *Journal of Personality and Social Psychology*, 44(1), pp. 113–126.

Devereaux, C. (2012) 'Moving into relationships: Dance/movement therapy with children with autism', in L. Gallo-Lopez and L.C. Rubin (eds.) *Play-based interventions for children and adolescents with autism spectrum disorders*. New York, NY: Routledge/Taylor & Francis Group, Vol. 72, pp. 105–120.

Eberhard-Kächele, M. (2010) 'Spiegelungsphänomene in der Tanztherapie/Körperpsychotherapie [Mirroring Phenomena in DMT / Body Psychotherapy]', in S. Bender (ed.) *Bewegungsanalyse von Interaktion–Movement Analysis of Interaction*. Berlin: Logos, pp. 193–212.

Eberhard-Kächele, M. (2012) 'Body memory, metaphor, and mirroring in movement therapy with trauma patients', in S.C. Koch, T. Fuchs, M. Summa, S. Ladewig and C. Müller (eds.) *Body Memory, Metaphor and Movement*. Philadelphia, PA: John Benjamins, pp. 267–287.

Feniger-Schaal, R., Hart, Y., Lotan, N., Koren-Karie, N. and Noy, L. (2018) 'The body speaks: Using the mirror game to link attachment and non-verbal behavior', *Frontiers in Psychology*, 9. 10.3389/fpsyg.2018.01560

Fischman, D. (2008) 'Therapeutic relationships and kinesthetic empathy', in S. Chaiklin and H. Wengrover (eds.) *Life is Dance: The art and science of dance therapy*. New York: Routledge, pp. 33–54.

Fraenkel, D.L. (1983) 'The relationship of empathy in movement to synchrony, echoing, and empathy in verbal interactions', *American Journal of Dance Therapy*, 6, pp. 31–48.

Fuchs, T. (2012) 'The phenomenology of body memory', in S. Koch, T. Fuchs, M. Summa, M. and C. Müller (eds.) *Body memory, metaphor and movement*. Amsterdam: John Benjamins, pp. 9–22.

Fuchs, T. and Koch, S.C. (2014) 'Embodied affectivity: On moving and being moved', *Frontiers in Psychology*, 5, p. 508, doi: 10.3389/fpsyg.2014.00508.

Gallagher, S. (2004) 'Understanding interpersonal problems in autism: Interaction theory as an alternative to theory of mind', *Philosophy, Psychiatry, & Psychology*, 11(3), pp. 199–217.

Gallagher, S. (2007) 'Simulation trouble', *Soc. Neuroscience*, 2, pp. 353–365. doi: 10.1080/17470910601183549.

García-Pérez, R.M., Lee, A. and Hobson, R.P. (2007) 'On intersubjective engagement in autism: A controlled study of nonverbal aspects of conversation', *Journal of Autism and Developmental Disorders*, 37(7), pp. 1310–1322.

Hatfield, E., Cacioppo, J.T. and Rapson, R.L. (1994) *Emotional contagion* (1. published ed.). Cambridge MA: Cambridge University Press.

Hildebrandt, M., Koch, S. and Fuchs, T. (2016) '"We dance and find each other": Effects of dance/movement therapy on negative symptoms in autism spectrum disorder', *Behavioral Sciences*, 6(4), p. 24. 10.3390/bs6040024

Husserl, E. (1952) *Ideen zu einer reinen Phänomenologie und phänomenologischen Philosophie [Ideen II; Husserliana IV]*. Den Haag: Martinus Nijhoff.

Hutto, D.D. (2007) 'The narrative practice hypothesis: Origins and applications to folk psychology', *Royal Institute of Philosophy*. Suppl. 60, pp. 43–68. doi:10.101 7/s1358246107000033.

Kestenberg, J.S. (1975) *Parents and children*. New York: Jason Aronson.

Kestenberg, J.S. and Sossin, K.M. (1979) *The role of movement pattems in developement* (Vol. 2). New York: Dance Notation Bureau.

Kestenberg Amighi, J., Loman, S., Lewis, P. and Sossin, K.M. (1999) *The meaning of movement: development and clinical perspectives of the kestenberg movement profile*. New York: Brunner-Routledge.

Klinger, L.G. and Williams, A. (2009) 'Cognitive behavioral interventions for students with autism spectrum disorders', in M.J. Mayer, R. Van Acker, J.E. Lochman and F.M. Gresham (eds.) *Cognitive behavioral interventions for students with emotional/behavioral disorders*. New York: Guilford Press, pp. 328–362.

Koch, S.C. (2020) 'Indications and contraindications in dance movement therapy: Learning from practitioner's experience', *GMS Journal of Arts Therapies*, 2(1). doi: 10.3205/jat000006

Koch, S.C., Mehl, L., Sobanski, E., Sieber, M. and Fuchs, T. (2015) 'Fixing the mirrors. A feasibility study of the effects of dance movement therapy on young adults with autism spectrum disorder', *Autism*, 19(3), pp. 338–350. doi: 10.11 77/1362361314522353. Epub 2014 Feb 24.

Koch, S.C., Riege, R.F.F., Tisborn, K., Biondo, J., Martin, L. and Beelmann, A. (2019) 'Effects of dance movement therapy and dance on health-related psychological outcomes. A meta-analysis update', *Frontiers in Psychology*, 10, p. 1806. doi: 10.3389/fpsyg.2019.01806

Kupfer, J., Brosig, B. and Brähler, E. (2001) *Toronto-Alexithymie-Skala-26 (TAS-26) - Deutsche Version. Manual*. Göttingen: Hogrefe.

Manders, E., Goodill, S., Koch, S.C., Giarelli, E., Polansky, M., Fisher, K. and Fuchs, T. (2021) 'The mirroring dance: Synchrony and interaction quality of five adolescents and adults on the autism spectrum in dance/movement therapy', *Frontiers in Psychology*, 12. 10.3389/fpsyg.2021.717389

Mastrominico, A., Fuchs, T., Manders, E., Steffinger, L., Hirjak, D., Sieber, M., Thomas, E., Holzinger, A., Konrad, A., Bopp, N. and Koch, S. (2018) 'Effects of dance movement therapy on adult patients with autism spectrum disorder: A randomized controlled trial', *Behavioral Sciences*, 8(7), p. 61. 10.3390/ bs8070061

McGarry, L.M. and Russo, F.A. (2011) 'Mirroring in dance/movement therapy: Potential mechanisms behind empathy enhancement', *The Arts in Psychotherapy*, 38(3), pp. 178–184.

Merleau-Ponty, M. (1962) *Phenomenology of perception*. London: Routledge & Kegan Paul.

Miles, L.K., Nind, L.K. and Macrea, C.N. (2009) 'The rhythm of rapport: Interpersonal synchrony and social perception', *Journal of Experimental Social Psychology*, 45 (3), pp. 585–589.

Mundy, P., Gwaltney, M. and Henderson, H. (2010) 'Self-referenced processing, neurodevelopment and joint attention in autism'. *Autism*, 14(5), pp. 408–429. doi: 10.1177/1362361310366315.

Nemetz, L. (2006) 'Moving with meaning: The historical progression of dance/movement therapy', in S.L. Brooke (Ed.) *Creative arts therapies manual: A guide to the history, theoretical approaches, assessment, and work with special populations of art, play, dance, music, drama, and poetry therapies.* Springfield: Charles C Thomas, pp. 95–108.

Nichols, E. (2019) *Moving blind spots: Cultural bias in the movement repertoire of dance/ movement therapists.* Expressive Therapies Capstone Theses. p. 150. https://digitalcommons.lesley.edu/expressive_theses/150

Paulus, C. (2009) *Der Saarbrücker Persönlichkeitsfragebogen SPF(IRI) zur Messung von Empathie.* Retreived 9 September 2012 from http://psydok.sulb.uni-saarland.de/volltexte/2009/2363.

Ramachandran, V.S. and Oberman, L.M. (2006) 'Broken mirrors: A theory of autism', *Scientific American*, 295(5), pp. 62–69.

Ramsayer, F. and Tschacher, W. (2011) 'Nonverbal synchrony in psychotherapy: Coordinated body-movement reflects relationship quality and outcome', *Journal of Consulting and Clinical Psychology*, 79(3), pp. 284–295.

Reichow, B. and Volkmar, F.R. (2010) 'Social skills interventions for individuals with autism: Evaluation for evidence-based practices within a best evidence synthesis framework', *Journal of Autism and Developmental Disorders*, 40(2), pp. 149–166.

Rizzolatti, G., Fadiga, L., Gallese, V. and Fogassi, L. (1996) 'Premotor cortex and the recognition of motor actions', *Cognitive Brain Research*, 3(2), pp. 131–141.

Rogers, C.R. (Ed.). (1951) *Client-centered therapy: Its current practice, implications, and theory.* Cambridge, MA: Houghton Mifflin.

Sandel, S.L. (1993) 'The process of empathic reflection in dance therapy', in S. Sandel, S. Chaiklin and A. Lohn (eds.) *Foundations of dance/movement therapy: The life and work of Marian Chace.* Columbia, MD: American Dance Therapy Association (ADTA).

Sandel, S.L., Chaiklin, S. and Lohn, A. (1993) *Foundations of dance/movement therapy: The life and work of Marian Chace.* Columbia, MD: American Dance Therapy Association (ADTA).

Savage, K.R., Dziobek, I., Teague, E.B. and Borod, J.C. (2010) *A new measure of empathy: Psychometric characteristics of the cognitive and emotional empathy questionnaire (CEEQ).* Unpublished Manuscript.

Schore, A. (1994) *Affect regulation and the origin of the self: The neurobiology of emotional development.* Hillsdale, New Jersey: Lawrence Erlbaum.

Schott-Billmann, F. (2015) *Primitive expression and dance therapy: When dancing heals.* London: Routledge.

Shai, D. and Belsky, J. (2011) 'When words just won't do: Introducing parental embodied mentalizing', *Child Development Perspectives*, 5, pp. 173–180.

Shuper-Engelhard, E. (2019) 'Embodying the couple relationship: Kinesthetic empathy and somatic mirroring in couples therapy', *Journal of Couple and Relationship Therapy*, 18(2), pp. 126–147. 10.1080/15332691.2018.1481801

Sinigaglia, C. (2009) Mirror in action. *Journal of Consciousness Studies*, 16, pp. 309–334.

Skoldberg, K. and Alvesson, M. (2000) *Reflexive methodology: New vistas for qualitative research*. United Kingdom: SAGE Publications.

Sodian, B. (2005) *Kognitive Entwicklung in der Kindheit. [Cognitive Development in Childhood.]* Stuttgart: Kohlhammer.

Stern, D. (2010) *Forms of vitality: Exploring dynamic experience in psychology, the arts, psychotherapy, and development*. Oxford: Oxford University Press.

Sullivan, H.S. (1953) *The interpersonal theory of psychiatry*. New York: Norton.

Tortora, S. (2005) *Dancing dialogue: Using the communicative power of movement with young children*. New York: Brooks Publishing (ISBN: 978-1-55766-834-9).

Trevarthen, C. (2004) *Learning about ourselves from children: Why a growing human brain needs interesting companions*. Retrieved 14 December 2009, from http://www.perception-in-action.ed.ac.uk/publications.htm

Chapter 8

# Interpersonal Art Psychotherapy for Adults with Autism and Intellectual Disabilities Being Treated in Secure Care

## A Single Case Study

*Simon S. Hackett*

## Introduction

### Neurodivergence in the Criminal Justice System

Whilst people who have autism do commit crimes and criminal offences it is also worth noting that people with autism are also more often victims of crimes rather than perpetrators (Gomez de la Cuesta, Taylor and Breckon, 2018). There is no evidence that people with autism commit crime at a higher rate than people in the general population (Gomez de la Cuesta et al., 2018) but people with autism do encounter the criminal justice system.

People who have additional needs associated with neurodivergence are currently seen to be disadvantaged during each stage of the criminal justice system, from arrest to detention and release. This has led to some consideration being given to the specific requirements and adjustments needed within the criminal justice system for people with autism and a range of neurodevelopmental conditions (Taylor et al., 2021).

### Adapting Psychological Therapies for People Who Have Autism, a Learning Disability, and/or Both

Practice guidelines have been agreed by clinical consensus in the UK for people with learning disabilities (Hackett et al., 2017 a). For people who have a learning disability and mental health problems, adaptations to psychological therapies can be important. This may mean agreeing intervention goals, developing an understanding of how the person expresses or describes their emotions, agreeing the structure, frequency, duration, content, and timing of the intervention, mode and pace of delivery, the level of flexibility needed, and how progress will be measured (e.g., visual representation of distress or wellbeing) (NICE, 2016).

DOI: 10.4324/9781003201656-11

Key recommendations for the delivery of psychological therapies for people who have autism include providing clear examples and using unambiguous language, slowing down the pace of the session, and using a more concrete and structured approach (The National Autistic Society UK, 2021). Additional considerations for people with autism might include making sure the therapy room is not overwhelming, using simple, plain language, giving time for people to process information and to answer questions, asking people if they would like someone close to them to support the sessions, helping people to label their own feelings and emotions, trying to integrate people's interests into the session if this is helpful, and noting down what you have covered so that you can share this with the person with autism (The National Autistic Society UK, 2021). For example, in inter-personal art psychotherapy, the therapist 'annotates' in writing or drawings for the client to help aid communication and understanding.

## Study Approach

In this chapter, an illustrative single-case study is presented. Components of interpersonal art psychotherapy are described and explained, with examples taken from Kyle's therapy sessions based upon contemporaneous/in-therapy audio-recordings. 'Kyle', was a Black British man in his late 20s with autism and a learning disability who was receiving treatment within a secure hospital. Repeated observation was used, including the Working Alliance Inventory-Therapist (Short Form) (WAI-T) (Munder et al., 2010) which was completed by the therapist after the first session and then every three weeks until 15 sessions had been completed. WAI-T total scores can range from 12 to 84 with higher scores reflecting more positive ratings of working alliance.

Motivation to participate in each therapy session was assessed via therapist observation rating using the Creative Arts Therapies Session Rating Scale (CAT-SRS) (Hackett, 2016 a). The CAT-SRS includes observational descriptors within four areas: (a) 'Communication: Use of the person's primary method of communicating: i.e., verbal language, nonverbal signs/gestures and vocalisations'; (b) 'Social skills: Use of listening, turn-taking, eye contact, appropriate body language, tone of voice'; (c) 'Motivation/participation: Motivation to engage actively throughout the session'; and (d) 'Linking: Ability to make links between personal experience and material that arises in therapy'.

Validated self-report outcome measures were completed by Kyle pre-therapy, post-therapy, and 12 weeks following the end of therapy. The Glasgow Anxiety Scale for people with intellectual disability (GAS-ID) (Mindham and Espie, 2003) is a 27-item self-rating scale of anxiety-symptoms for people who have a mild intellectual disability. Higher scores indicate higher levels of anxiety with the maximum possible score on this scale being 54. There are also subtotals for 'worries', 'fears' and 'physiological symptoms'. The Brief Symptom Inventory (BSI) (Derogatis, 1993) is a 53-item self-report inventory with sub-items that can be calculated for a Global Severity Index (GSI), Positive Symptom Total (PST), and Positive Symptom Distress Index (PSDI). Higher scores in this measure also indicate higher, and more clinically prevalent, psychiatric symptoms.

For the purposes of this illustrative case study, Kyle's individual GAS-ID and BSI scores have been analysed in comparison with the pre-therapy scores from his fellow participants ($n$ = 19) recruited to the interpersonal art psychotherapy feasibility study (Hackett et al., 2020). A comparison has been calculated using a web-based programme 'Singlims.exe' (Crawford and Garthwaite, 2002) to show the percentage of Kyle's peers (the normal population/norm or control sample) falling below his score, as an indicator of improvement or deterioration against this peer group during the period. An effect size is also indicated, which can be applied in single case-design (Hackett and Aafjes-van Doorn, 2019), as a measure of the magnitude and impact of the intervention, shown in the difference between means and expressed in standard deviation units (Kazdin, 2011).

### Interpersonal Art Psychotherapy

Interpersonal art psychotherapy consisted of 15 individual weekly one-hour sessions. It is currently being provided by UK Health and Care Professions Council (HCPC) registered Art Psychotherapists with experience of working in secure care.

Interpersonal art psychotherapy uses a structured manualised approach that has been developed following single-case design research on art psychotherapy in secure care for people with autism, intellectual disabilities, and/or both (Hackett, 2012). The results of these initial single-case design studies highlighted components of treatment that could be associated with helpful outcomes for each participant. For example, one case of a man with autism highlighted that artwork produced within the therapy helped to facilitate discussion about his sexual fantasies and risks to others as part of treatment in a secure care setting (Hackett, 2016 b). A psychodynamic approach within art psychotherapy has also been shown to help a patient with anti-social personality disorder develop more positive interpersonal interactions with staff and family members (Hackett and Aafjes-van Doorn, 2019). Further feasibility work showed that participants ($n$ = 17) who completed 15 sessions of interpersonal art psychotherapy had lower rates of verbal aggression and reported a reduction in personal distress related to their psychiatric symptoms (Hackett et al., 2020).

Aims of interpersonal art psychotherapy and components (in brief) (see also Table 8.1):

- To address the clients immediate (1) concerns/distress or problems. To develop these into person centred therapy goals and encourage the use of (2) positive coping responses and self-management skills.

*Table 8.1* Interpersonal art psychotherapy component descriptors

| Comp. | Session/s | Descriptor | Artmaking |
|---|---|---|---|
| 1. | 1 | **Establishing person centred therapy goals:** The client is asked about three things that they would like to see improve or achieve. Goals are rated on a five-point scale with the anchor points 'the worst it could be' to 'the best it could be'. Therapy goals are reviewed with the therapist and scored by the client again in all subsequent therapy sessions. | Draw a picture of something you like |
| 2. | 2 to 3 | **Positive coping responses and self-management techniques:** Coping responses in interpersonal art psychotherapy focus on utilising the clients existing strengths, knowledge, interests, and their willingness to try out new approaches to developing positive coping responses. The client is asked to draw a picture of themselves at a time when they are feeling happy and/or relaxed, leading into a conversation with the therapist about what they usually do to cope and self-manage. | Draw ways you find it helpful to relax |
| 3. | 4 to 5 | **Relationships:** Work on relationships highlight how the client sees other people in their life, how they think other people see them, and the kind of things they want to get out of their different relationships. The client is asked to draw out a simple picture of people they know. This information is recorded or annotated by the therapist and contributes towards the development of a 'shared understanding', component 5. | Draw people you know |
| 4. | 6 to 10 | **Personal Events:** The client is asked to complete a drawing of an event that can be discussed. This is introduced as 'things that have happened in your life in the past or recently, in the last few weeks'. Both positive and negatively perceived events can be drawn by the client. The event pictures provide a visual record that is personally generated by the client and associated with a specific conversation with the therapist. Discussion of events can provide additional contextual information about events that have taken place in the participants' life. Additional questions can include 'what made you choose to draw this event' and 'what do you think about this event now?' | Draw an event that has happened |
| 5. | 11 to 12 | **Building a shared understanding:** For a shared understanding to be developed between the client and the therapist a working therapeutic alliance is required. Developing and agreeing a shared formulation about interpersonal styles of | Shared completion of a worksheet |

(Continued)

*Table 8.1* (Continued)

| Comp. | Session/s | Descriptor | Artmaking |
|---|---|---|---|
| | | interacting is based upon integrating or linking the four previous components (1. therapy goals; 2. positive coping responses; 3. relationships; and 4. events). Conversation in the session can be captured using an interpersonal art psychotherapy worksheet that has been designed to help gather key points from the topics and material generated by the client in previous sessions. | |
| **6.** | *13 to 14* | **Imagined future:** This component allows the client to identify their own wishes and needs for the future with a view to enabling them to become motivated to make changes that help them maintain progress. The client is asked to draw a picture of themselves in the future and discuss the content of the picture with the therapist. The client's perceptions of themselves in the future are allowed to be aspirational. The rationale for this approach is to encourage motivation about how the client sees their future and their progress. | Draw a picture of yourself in the future |
| **7.** | *15* | **Therapy review and close:** To end the therapy the therapist leads a review of the drawings that have been made and asks the client to identify their most important artwork/s. The client also has an opportunity to write a letter to people about their progress in therapy, for example to their responsible clinician, the multi-disciplinary team in secure care, or someone they are close to. The client leaves therapy with a simple personalised summary in a letter from the therapist outlining the therapy components they have worked through together. | Chose the most important artwork/s that you have made |

- To identify 'themes' and 'patterns' that perpetuate 'styles' of interacting with others that are problematic. These themes are discovered through conversations linked to guided drawing tasks on (3) relationships and (4) events.
- To use agreed themes as the basis of forming a (5) 'shared understanding' with the client about areas that can change to reduce the impact of personal 'styles' of interacting with others and patterns of thinking, coping, and responding to others that might perpetuate interpersonal difficulties.
- To enable the client to become motivated to make changes that help them progress towards their (6) imagined future.
- To (7) review and close the work positively in a way that the client can continue to improve or maintain their progress.

## The Therapeutic Approach

Therapists are given training and guidance about how to conduct inter-personal art psychotherapy sessions and are asked to 'avoid making assumptions', but rather to check things out with the client through questioning and to inquire about what the client has meant by the words they use. Similarly, therapists are asked to 'avoid making interpretations and speculating', for example, not interpreting perceived 'hidden', 'symbolic', and 'unspoken' meanings. Speculation about what the client has or has not said or implied in their words is instead replaced by giving the client feedback about what has been understood and asking about areas related to the interpersonal art psychotherapy components and tasks. A technique of 'annotating' the client's words by writing them down during the session or drawing a diagram or picture is used by the therapist. These approaches are intended to build the clients confidence that they are being understood by the therapists and support communication.

Qualified art psychotherapists (to UK Masters level) who completed two days of training and familiarisation with the therapy manual, including formal teaching, group discussion and rehearsal/role-play, alongside fortnightly clinical supervision, achieved close adherence and fidelity to the directions given in the therapy manual (82%) (Hackett et al., 2020). In a post-study focus group, the art psychotherapists who delivered inter-personal art psychotherapy reflected that the participants with autism completed all planned sessions. This was notable because within their normal clinical practice, often using a less structured approach, their experience was that people with autism sometimes chose to end therapy early.

The theoretical model underpinning interpersonal art psychotherapy is based on research carried out using the Core Conflictual Relationship Theme (CCRT) (L. Luborsky, 1994; Luborsky and Crits-Cristoph, 2003). This model comprises three common elements seen in the clients reporting of interactions observed in studies of psychodynamic psychotherapy (Luborsky, 2003). Within interpersonal art psychotherapy, the therapist is asked to 'tune into' visual and verbal material from the client about their relationships. Interactions within relationships are then considered from three perspectives.

- Wish = the needs or intention of the client.
- Other's responses = other people's responses (imagined or actual) to the client.
- Self-responses = the client's own responses (imagined or actual).

This interpersonal relationship model can be applied from the beginning to the end of interpersonal art psychotherapy. Using guided artmaking tasks and specific questions, the art psychotherapist seeks to find out about the clients' wishes or needs in relation to their interactions with others, such as what they had wanted or hoped for from the interaction and what they say about the other person responding to them. This approach cuts across all seven therapy components (see Table 8.1).

In interpersonal art psychotherapy, drawings by clients can be very simple (e.g., line drawings, stick figures). However, if clients want to use a wider range of materials to make detailed and rich images this is also encouraged. Whilst a range of art making equipment and materials can be used, depending upon what is available and what is safely permitted in the secure setting, interpersonal art psychotherapy can be successful with a limited range of art materials. The basic art materials required are felt tip pens and/ or pencils and A4/A3 size white paper.

## A Selected Illustrative Case Study of the Components of Interpersonal Art Psychotherapy

'Kyle', a Black British man in his late 20s with autism and a learning disability, was recruited to a randomised controlled feasibility study of interpersonal art psychotherapy (Hackett et al., 2017 b, 2020). Kyle had been convicted of a criminal sexual assault offence and was being treated in a NHS medium secure hospital in London, UK. He had been in secure care for six years and volunteered to take part in the research study which randomised participants to either interpersonal art psychotherapy and usual care or a usual care waiting list. Prior to being in the secure hospital Kyle had spent time in prison and had been placed in foster care during periods of his childhood. He had additional mental health diagnoses of paranoid schizophrenia and antisocial personality disorder. Kyle completed 15 therapy sessions of one-to-one interpersonal art psychotherapy.

**Component 1.** Establishing therapy goals
   *Personcentred goals were established at the start of therapy and agreed between Kyle and his therapist (Table 8.2).*

Table 8.2 Kyle's therapy goals

| Kyle's therapy goals | at therapy start | at therapy end |
|---|---|---|
| 'I get bothered when people talk about my weight and food portions' | 'not so good' | 'good' |
| 'I am struggling with my physical health and it makes me feel angry' | 'OK' | 'good' |
| 'It bothers me when I fall asleep in meetings' | 'not so good' | 'good' |

Note: responses can be 1='the worst it can be'; 2='not so good'; 3='OK'; 4='good'; 5='the best it can be'.

*In early therapy sessions Kyle spoke of his concerns about his body-image, weight manage-ment, and physical health. Kyle rated his therapy goals as having improved at the end of therapy.*

## Component 2. Positive coping responses and self-management techniques

*Kyle identified positive coping responses that he found helpful; these were listening to music, watching TV, talking to others and speaking to support and nursing staff at the hospital, resting, going to his room to calm down and/or sleep, reading, cooking and eating food, and playing computer games. Kyle also thought that he could try out doing a bit more exercise by going to the gym and joining a walking group when it was available. He also said that he wanted to try to get some work experience in the future.*

## Component 3. Relationships

*Kyle drew a picture of himself, his mother and father (Figure 8.1), and a comedian he had seen at a live performance. At this point in therapy Kyle did not identify or speak about other relationships, friendships, or about interactions with people around him, such as support or nursing staff in the secure hospital. Kyle did give some examples of times he spent with his mum, such as going to church together and eating meals together, and being with his father, com-menting that he liked his father, saying 'he gives me money'.*

## Component 4. Personal Events

*Kyle was able to identify and draw five events that were significant to him. Kyle's chosen events ranged from the day before one of his therapy sessions, when he was given feedback about his physical health status, something that concerned him a great deal. He said that he felt upset with the doctor who told him about his raised blood pressure. Kyle's body image and weight management was a concern at the start of therapy and something he wanted to see improve as a personal therapy goal. Kyle also became upset and angry with staff when they tried to speak to him about his health and diet, impacting negatively upon his relationships and his mood. Kyle responded to this event by saying that he wanted to do something about it and understood it was serious, which generated further discussion in the therapy about what he thought he could do.*

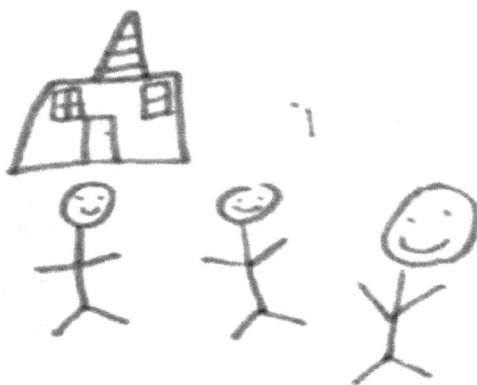

*Figure 8.1* Family, Mum, Dad and Kyle

*Kyle spoke about one early adverse event when he was a child and he witnessed two people having sexual intercourse. He said, 'A child should not see that sort of thing'. Kyle had also been convicted of sexual offences and had been assessed as having risky behaviour related to sexual assaults on others. This also formed a significant part of his work with the therapist in sessions and more generally in his risk-management and treatment within secure care.*

*Kyle recalled times that he said were good events, such as going to a church and being at a large religious gathering at an arena. Kyle also gave an account of an event that he had mixed feelings about when he had spent time playing on computer games with two friends who were the same age as him, when he was in his early 20s. Shortly after this Kyle went to prison and he missed seeing them. He then described this as 'not good', and said that when he thought about this now he was 'sad, not happy' and 'embarrassed'.*

## Component 5. Building a shared understanding

*As well as listing Kyle's therapy goals, positive coping responses, relationships, and events, a shared understanding was reached between Kyle and his therapist. They recognised that (interpersonally) Kyle could get on with people but that he could also be 'hostile, to get what I want', that he could be 'powerful and can scare people if I get angry'. Kyle said that he had committed offences and that he had been in trouble with the police and that he had also been a victim of others.*

## Component 6. Imagined future

*In the future, Kyle said that he wanted to learn to live independently, 'to live life'. Kyle said that he needed to change some of his behaviours and mentioned changing his eating patterns and doing more exercise.*

## Component 7. Therapy review and close

*At the end of therapy, comments by his therapist, his secure care multi-disciplinary team, and Kyle's own accounts indicated that he made noticeable improvements, such as:*

- *Being able to talk to staff with whom he had previously found it difficult to work.*
- *Appearing to be more positive and feeling that he was receiving a more positive response from others. This was also related to Kyle making efforts to work with staff more constructively to help manage his own weight (a therapy goal).*
- *Becoming more engaged with members of his multi-disciplinary team in secure care, being more open in the discussion, more cooperative, having less conflict, and less anger when discussing staff support for his weight management.*
- *The change was noted by his therapist, who concluded that Kyle had shifted towards being more open and engaged and able to take on board other people's point of view.*

## Findings

### Therapeutic Alliance and Motivation to Engage in Therapy

Kyle's total working alliance (WAI-T) scores ranged from being highest in week three (63), to lowest in week six (37), with scores rising again in the following and final therapy session (54). Mean scores from six observations (Mean = 55.16: Standard Deviation = 9.38) indicate relatively high working alliance throughout therapy with a recovery in alliance following a reduced alliance score being observed during one session in the therapy.

Motivation to participate in sessions was assessed via therapist observation rating using the Creative Arts Therapies Session Rating Scale (CAT-SRS) (Hackett, 2016 a). Kyle was rated as having high motivation throughout therapy. The observation descriptor being chosen by the therapist in his first session was 'motivated to participate most of the time. When prompting is required responds to the first prompt given'. For the remainder of the therapy the descriptor chosen was 'motivated all of the time to actively participate throughout'.

### Anxiety and Psychological Distress

Kyle completed assessments at pre-therapy, post-therapy, and at 12 weeks follow-up. Kyle's response to interpersonal art psychotherapy is shown predominantly in measures of anxiety (GAS-ID worries) and distress related to his psychiatric symptoms (Brief Symptom Inventory-Positive Symptom Distress index (BSI-PSDI) (see Table 8.3).

At the 12-week follow-up, a medium to large effect size (ES) can be seen for GAS-ID worries (ES = –0.76) with just 23.15% of Kyle's peers (Estimated percentage of norm/normal population falling below case's score), as compared to 88.62% pre-therapy.

Kyle also makes notable improvement on the PSDI (ES =1.89) with just 4.03% of his peers falling below his score at follow-up as compared to 64.46% pre-therapy. Total BSI scores above 64 are within the clinical range for people with learning disabilities in secure care (Kellett et al., 2003). Kyle's BSI total score moves from being within this clinical range at pre-assessment (67) to below the clinical range post-therapy (47) with further improvement at follow-up (33). This is a positive measurable clinical indicator of improvement in Kyle's mental health anxiety and personal distress following completion of interpersonal art psychotherapy.

### Discussion

People with autism who are assessed as not coping in prison or who have needs that are seen to be better met within the health service are sometimes referred or transferred to secure care. Interpersonal art psychotherapy has been designed as a structured and manualised approach for people who have autism, a learning disability, or both (Hackett et al., 2020). The approach used within this therapy draws from research developed with people who have a range of mental health difficulties (Hackett, Porter and Taylor, 2013; Hackett, 2016 b; Hackett et al., 2017 b, 2020; Hackett and Aafjes-van Doorn, 2019) including those who have conditions broadly considered

Table 8.3 Kyle's scores compared to his peers (normal population/norm/control sample)

| Measure / Item | Pre-Therapy | | | Post-Therapy | | | Follow-up (12 weeks) | | |
|---|---|---|---|---|---|---|---|---|---|
| | Score t value (Significance test on difference between case's score and control sample) | Effect Size for difference between case and controls (95% CI) | Estimated percentage of normal population falling below case's score (95% Lower to Upper CI) | Score t value | Effect Size (95% CI) | Estimated percentage of norm (95% Lower to Upper CI) | Score t value | Effect Size (95% CI) | Estimated percentage of norm (95% Lower to Upper CI) |
| GAS-ID Total | 29    0.81 | 0.83 (0.30 to 1.34) | 78.63% (61.80% to 91.14%) | 22    0.10 | 0.10 (−0.34 to 0.55) | 53.98% (36.38% to 71.00%) | 18    0.40 | 0.41 (−0.05 to 0.88) | 65.52% (47.68% to 81.08%) |
| GAS-ID Worries | 16    1.25 | 1.28 (0.66 to 1.88) | 88.62% (74.54% to 97.02%) | 10    0.25 | −0.25 (−0.71 to 0.20) | 40.27% (23.87% to 58.09%) | 8    −0.75 | −0.76 (−1.27 to −0.24) | 23.15% (10.11% to 40.25%) |
| GAS-ID Specific fears | 6    0.34 | 0.35 (−0.11 to 0.81) | 63.20% (45.34% to 79.12%) | 4    −0.18 | −0.18 (−0.64 to 0.26) | 42.78% (26.09% to 60.53%) | 4    −0.18 | −0.18 (−0.64 to 0.26) | 42.78% (26.09% to 60.53%) |
| GAS-ID Physiological symptoms | 7    0.23 | 0.24 (−0.21 to 0.69) | 59.16% (41.36% to 75.63%) | 8    0.57 | 0.58 (0.09 to 1.06) | 71.25% (53.65% to 85.71%) | 6    −0.10 | −0.10 (−0.55 to 0.34) | 46.04% (29.01% to 63.64%) |
| BSI Total | 67    0.37 | 0.38 (−0.08 to 0.84) | 64.46% (46.60% to 80.18%) | 47    −0.30 | −0.30 (−0.76 to 0.15) | 38.32% (22.18% to 56.17%) | 33    −0.77 | −0.79 (−1.30 to −0.27) | 22.38% (9.56% to 39.37%) |
| BSI – Global Severity Index (GSI) | 1.27    0.42 | 0.43 (−0.04 to 0.90) | 66.21% (48.38% to 81.65%) | 0.89    −0.24 | −0.25 (−0.70 to 0.20) | 40.34% (23.93% to 58.16%) | 0.63    −0.70 | −0.72 (−1.22 to −0.21) | 24.37% (10.98% to 41.62%) |

(Continued)

Table 8.3 (Continued)

| Measure / Item | Pre-Therapy | | | | Post-Therapy | | | | Follow-up (12 weeks) | | | |
|---|---|---|---|---|---|---|---|---|---|---|---|---|
| | Score | t value Significance test on difference between case's score and control sample | Effect Size for difference between case and controls (95% CI) | Estimated percentage of normal population falling below case's score (95% Lower to Upper CI) | Score | t value | Effect Size (95% CI) | Estimated percentage of norm (95% Lower to Upper CI) | Score | t value | Effect Size (95% CI) | Estimated percentage of norm (95% Lower to Upper CI) |
| BSI – Positive Symptom Total (PST) | 41 | 1.49 | 1.53 (0.85 to 2.19) | 92.39% (80.35% to 98.59%) | 32 | 0.69 | 0.70 (0.19 to 1.20) | 75.09% (57.79% to 88.62%) | 25 | 0.06 | 0.06 (−0.38 to 0.51) | 52% (35.07% to 69.74%) |
| BSI – Positive Symptom Distress Index (PSDI) | 1.64 | 0.37 | 0.38 (−0.08 to 0.84) | 64.46% (46.60% to 80.18%) | 1.47 | −1.84 | −1.89 (−2.64 to −1.12) | 4.07% (0.40 to 13.06%) | 1.33 | −1.85 | −1.89 (−2.65 to −1.12) | 4.03% (0.40% to 12.98%) |

Note: Normal population/control sample n=19 (Hackett et al., 2020). GAS-ID = Glasgow Anxiety Scale-ID (Mindham & Espie, 2003) clinical cut-off = 15; BSI = Brief Symptom Inventory (Derogatis, 1993) clinical cut-off = 64 (Kellet et al., 2003); CI=Confidence Interval.

within the criminal justice system as neurodivergent and therefore requiring system level adaptation at every stage (Taylor et al., 2021).

Adapting psychological therapies for people with autism and/or a learning disability is important and a set of clear recommendations has been developed within the UK (NICE, 2016; The National Autistic Society UK, 2021), alongside specific art therapy guidance for people who have learning disabilities (Hackett et al., 2017 a). Whilst the current provision of interpersonal art psychotherapy described here has been tested within secure care, the structure approach that it uses aligns closely with these recommendations and could therefore be provided more widely to people who have autism accessing community-based services.

The illustrative case of Kyle, a man with autism, a learning disability, and additional mental health diagnosis, has been selected and reported here as a single case study (Kazdin, 2011) illustrative of specific components of interpersonal art psychotherapy. Helpful interpersonal outcomes have been reported from observations, in addition to Kyle's own reporting of improvement in his personal therapy goals. Comparative analysis against a normal population/control sample (Crawford and Garthwaite, 2002) has been carried out on validated self-report measures at pre-therapy, post-therapy, and at follow-up to identify additional helpful individual outcomes for Kyle. This provides a measurable clinical indication that reduced anxiety and improvement in personal distress related to mental health symptoms can be expected outcomes from interpersonal art psychotherapy with people who have autism.

### Conclusion

Whilst further work on assessing the effectiveness of manualised interpersonal art psychotherapy is needed, this approach and the components found within it fit closely with current recommendations for psychological therapies with people who have autism (The National Autistic Society UK, 2021). Interpersonal art psychotherapy now offers the potential for a widening of the psychological treatment choice available to people with autism who have mental health needs.

### Acknowledgements

I would like to thank Kate Rothwell, Head Art Psychotherapist, who provided interpersonal art psychotherapy to 'Kyle' and reviewed this chapter before publication. I would like to thank Kyle who was one of three participants with a diagnosis of autism who took part in a feasibility study of interpersonal art psychotherapy.

## Ethical Approval

NHS Health Research Authority (HRA) IRAS project ID 191223, Research Ethics Committee (REC) reference 16/NE/0220.

## References

Crawford, J.R. and Garthwaite, P.H. (2002) 'Investigation of the single case in neuropsychology: Confidence limits on the abnormality of test scores and test score differences', *Neuropsychologia*, 40(8), pp. 1196–1208. doi:10.1016/S0028-3932 (01)00224-X.

Derogatis, L.R. (1993) *Brief Symptom Inventory (BSI) administration, scoring, and procedures manual* (3rd edn.). Minneapolis: NCS Pearson, Inc.

Gomez de la Cuesta, G., Taylor, J.L. and Breckon, S.E. (2018) 'Autism spectrum disorders and offending behaviour', in W.R. Lindsay and J.L. Taylor (eds.) *The Wiley handbook on offenders with intellectual and developmental disabilities. Research, training, and practice*. Chichester: Wiley Blackwell, pp. 365–383.

Hackett. (2016a) 'The combined arts therapies team: Sharing practice development in the National Health Service in England', *Approaches: An Interdisciplinary Journal of Music Therapy*, 8(1), pp. 42–49.

Hackett, S. (2016b) 'Art Psychotherapy with an adult with autistic spectrum disorder and sexually deviant dreams: A single-case study including the client's responses to treatment', in K. Rothwell (ed.) *Forensic arts therapies: Anthology of practice and research*. London: Free Association Books Limited.

Hackett, S., Porter, J. and Taylor, J.L. (2013) 'The core conflictual relationship theme (CCRT) method: testing with adult offenders who have intellectual and developmental disabilities', *Advances in Mental Health and Intellectual Disability*, 7. doi: 10.1108/AMHID-06-2013-0039.

Hackett, S.S. (2012) *Art psychotherapy with adult offenders who have intellectual and developmental disabilities*. (PhD), University of Northumbria, Newcastle upon Tyne. Retrieved from http://nrl.northumbria.ac.uk/10354/1/hackett.simon_phd.pdf.

Hackett, S.S. (2016) 'Art psychotherapy with an adult with autistic spectrum disorder and sexually deviant dreams: A single-case study including the client's responses to treatment', in K. Rothwell (ed.) *Forensic arts therapies: Anthology of practice and research*. Free Association Books Limited.

Hackett, S.S. and Aafjes-van Doorn, K. (2019) 'Psychodynamic art psychotherapy for the treatment of aggression in an individual with antisocial personality disorder in a secure forensic hospital: A single-case design study', *Psychotherapy*, 56(2), pp. 297–308. doi:10.1037/pst0000232.

Hackett, S.S., Ashby, L., Parker, K., Goody, S. and Power, N. (2017a) 'UK art therapy practice-based guidelines for children and adults with learning disabilities', *International Journal of Art Therapy*, 22(2), pp. 84–94. doi:10.1080/17454832.2017.1319870.

Hackett, S.S., Taylor, J.L., Freeston, M., Jahoda, A., McColl, E., Pennington, L. and Kaner, E. (2017b) 'Interpersonal art psychotherapy for the treatment of aggression in people with learning disabilities in secure care: a protocol for a randomised controlled feasibility study', *Pilot and Feasibility Studies*, 3(1), p. 42. doi:10.1186/ s40814-017-0186-z.

Hackett, S.S., Zubala, A., Aafjes-van Doorn, K., Chadwick, T., Harrison, T.L., Bourne, J., ... Kaner, E. (2020) 'A randomised controlled feasibility study of interpersonal art psychotherapy for the treatment of aggression in people with intellectual disabilities in secure care', *Pilot and Feasibility Studies*, 6(1), p. 180. doi:10.1186/s40814-020-00703-0.

Kazdin, A.E. (2011) *Single-case research designs: Methods for clinical and applied settings* (2nd edn.). New York: Oxford University Press.

Kellett, S., Beail, N., Newman, D.W. and Frankish, P. (2003) 'Utility of the brief symptom inventory in the assessment of psychological distress', *Journal of Applied Research in Intellectual Disabilities*, 16(2), pp. 127–134.

Luborsky, L. (1994) 'The core conflictual relationship theme', *Psychotherapy Research*, 4. doi:10.1080/10503309412331334012.

Luborsky, L. (2003) 'The relationship anecdote paradigm (RAP) interview as a versatile source of narratives', in L. Luborsky and P. Crits-Christoph (eds.) *Understanding transference: The core conflictual relationship theme method* (2nd edn.). Washington: American Psychological Association, pp. 109–120.

Luborsky, L. and Crits-Cristoph, P. (2003) *Understanding transference: The core conflictual relationship theme method* (2nd edn.). Washington: American Psychological Association.

Mindham, J. and Espie, C.A. (2003) 'Glasgow anxiety scale for people with an Intellectual Disability (GAS-ID): Development and psychometric properties of a new measure for use with people with mild intellectual disability', *Journal of Intellectual Disability Research*, 47(1), pp. 22–30.

Munder, T., Wilmers, F., Leonhart, R., Linster, H.W. and Barth, J. (2010) 'Working alliance inventory-short revised (WAI-SR): Psychometric properties in outpatients and inpatients', *Clinical Psychology and Psychotherapy*, 17(3), pp. 231–239. doi:10. 1002/cpp.658.

NICE (2016) *Mental health problems in people with learning disabilities: prevention, assessment and management. (NICE Clinical Guideline NG54)*. London: National Institute for Health and Care Excellence.

Taylor, C., Russell, J. and Winsor, T. (2021) *Neurodiversity in the criminal justice system: A review of evidence*. Retrieved from https://www.justiceinspectorates.gov. uk/cjji/wp-content/uploads/sites/2/2021/07/Neurodiversity-evidence-review-web-2021.pdf.

The National Autistic Society UK. (2021) *Good practice guide for professionals delivering talking therapies for autistic adults and children*. Retrieved from https:// s2.chorus-mk.thirdlight.com/file/24/asDKIN9as.klK7easFDsalAzTC/NAS-Good-Practice-Guide-A4.pdf.

Chapter 9

# Parental Perceptions of the Process and Impact of Dramatherapy Group Sessions for Adolescents with Autism Spectrum Disorder

*Loukia Bololia*

## Introduction

Autism spectrum disorder (ASD) is a lifelong developmental condition with onset typically between one and two years of age, affecting ways of understanding, interacting and communicating with others as well as the processing of social and sensory experiences (American Psychiatric Association [APA], 2013). There are debates and different standpoints regarding the description, understanding and perception of ASD. Notably, there is a considerable heterogeneity of clinical characteristics in every individual and over the lifespan, which vary in severity level, clinical presentation and persistence into adulthood. As ASD diagnosis involves individuals with a broad range of features, with diverse strengths, abilities and difficulties, it is commonly agreed that there is not an 'one-size-fits-all' type of support. There is a need for beneficial therapeutic approaches that respect individuality, encompass subjective experiences, facilitate social connections and provide every individual with the means to reach their full potential (Fletcher-Watson and Happé, 2019). While it is still relatively limited, there is a growing body of research which contributes towards understanding how and why dramatherapy, a form of psychotherapy that intentionally uses drama and theatre-arts creative processes, can support children and young people with ASD. For instance, through engaging a plethora of art forms and drama techniques, such as symbolic work, role-playing, improvisations, enactments and stories, within the therapeutic encounter research findings have shown that dramatherapy can enhance social skills, relationship development and connection with others, empower confidence and improve motivation in school whilst reducing stressful feelings and externalising behaviour (Bololia et al., 2022; D'Amico et al., 2015; Godfrey and Haythorne, 2013; Wilmer-Barbrook, 2013). However, there is a need for further empirical research evidence in this field.

DOI: 10.4324/9781003201656-12

## Rationale and Importance of the Present Study

The present chapter presents the qualitative strand of a mixed-method evaluation study focused on the process and outcomes of 15 dramatherapy group sessions for adolescents, 11–17 years old, with an ASD diagnosis. This qualitative study aimed to address the research gap in the field by exploring parents/carers' unique observations and insights into the process and impact of dramatherapy group sessions for their adolescents. It is worth noting that adolescence is a sensitive transitional life period involving physical and psychosocial changes, identity development, maturation, integration into society and future planning. Thus, it is critical to conduct research on the efficacy of interventions and support approaches in the different developmental stages of individuals with ASD (Goldin and Matson, 2017). Having said that, adolescents are under-represented in ASD intervention research (Reichow et al., 2010). With regard to parental involvement, it has been posited that caregivers' contributions are of paramount importance in therapeutic interventions for children and adolescents with ASD (Burrell and Borrego, 2012). More importantly, in contrast to adult group therapy, the role of parents in children and adolescent group therapy can improve the therapeutic support (Haen and Aronson, 2017).

## Dramatherapy Group Sessions

Before presenting the research methods employed in this study, information regarding the structure and content of the sessions are offered. In total, 28 adolescents participated in seven dramatherapy groups with each group including three to seven members. All seven groups completed 15 weekly dramatherapy group sessions with a duration of 90 minutes each that took place in a private psychological therapy centre in Greece. The sessions were facilitated by qualified dramatherapists with professional experience working with people with ASD and supervised by a clinical supervisor. Dramatherapy frameworks and approaches involved the play-drama continuum entailing sensory-motor play, imitative play, pretend play, dramatic play, drama-roles (Jones, 2007), a developmental paradigm starting with embodiment work and projective play to role-taking (Jennings, 1999) and Chesner's (1995) multimodal framework for people with learning difficulties, integrating movement, music, games, role-playing and performance.

## Research Aim

The present study aimed at exploring parental views on the process and effects of 15 weekly dramatherapy group sessions for adolescents with an ASD diagnosis. The research question posed was the following: What are the parents/carers' perceptions about the process and impact of dramatherapy group sessions for their adolescents?

## Study Approach

This qualitative inquiry used face-to-face semi-structured interviews with one or both parents/carers after the completion of all sessions. Qualitative interviewing was employed as it is considered suitable for in-depth exploration of human experiences and meaning-making, as well as capturing process and outcomes of programmes involving individualised effects (Silverman, 2005).

### Participants

Within the context of this study, 23 mothers/carers and 16 fathers/carers of median age 46 and 50 years, respectively, participated in semi-structured interviews. Most participants were self-employed or employed in public and private sector. 35% of mothers/carers were either unemployed (26.1%) or retired (8.7%) and 12.5% of fathers/carers were retired. In addition, more than half of the female interviewees held an undergraduate degree whist approx. 26% had completed postgraduate studies. The relevant education level of the male participants stood at 69% and 12.5% for undergraduate and postgraduate studies, respectively.

### Procedure

#### Interview Structure and Process

Following the completion of all group sessions for adolescents, interviews with parents/carers were arranged. Overall, 25 interviews took place and each interview lasted 30–40 minutes. In a friendly and respectful manner, key questions were asked, exploring parental perspectives on potential positive or negative aspects or incidents, or behavioural or life changes, during or following the sessions. Also, any impact on family relationships or peer-school-community relationships were discussed.

### Ethical Considerations and Quality Review

This study was granted ethics approval by a Higher Education Research Ethics Committee. Informed consent was signed by the participants who were informed of the voluntary and free-of-charge nature of their participation. Anonymity and confidentiality were ensured, and any personal identifiers were removed from all interview records. While reporting the findings, parents/carers are not identified in text segments; instead, pseudonyms are used for everyone.

A fieldwork reflective journal (i.e., audit trail) was kept throughout the study by the researcher, ensuring transparency and rigour in the research process (Onwuegbuzie and Leech, 2007). Also, both the credibility and confirmability of findings were ensured by an independent qualitative researcher who participated in the coding process during data analysis. According to O'Connor and Joffe (2020), an independent reviewer typically codes 10%–25% of randomly selected data units. In the current study, a random number generator was used to select seven (28%) interview transcripts for coding by the independent qualitative researcher. The code patterns were then compared and where there were any discrepancies a mutual agreement was reached through discussion. Lastly, participant quotes are included in the findings, establishing trustworthiness and credibility through a vivid and faithful description (Saldaña, 2014).

## Analysis

Thematic analysis was employed as it is an appropriate analytic method for identifying patterns and themes occurring in qualitative data. It is also apposite for research questions focusing on participants' understanding, illuming diverse perspectives and unexpected insights (Clarke and Braun, 2018). Thematic analysis is a recursive process rather than a linear one, involving six stages: familiarisation with the data; coding; searching for themes; reviewing themes; defining and naming themes; writing-up. Each emerging theme could be considered as a 'key character in the story we are telling about the data' (Clarke and Braun, 2018, p. 108). The interview data were analysed, and seven overall themes were identified and displayed along with their corresponding subthemes (Figure 9.1).

## Results

### Fostering Socialisation

According to the caregivers' observations, their adolescents were offered an opportunity to explore relationship building and making friends within the safe environment of dramatherapy sessions. Friendships were developed, especially among adolescents sharing common hobbies or interests. This might be also viewed as a restorative or corrective emotional experience because most adolescents have reportedly been recipients of bullying behaviour from peers.

> He is bullied at school because he has a shadow teacher. He was constantly speaking about other members of the group, calling them 'my friends'. (Peter)
> He does not have any other friends and he made a good friend during the group meetings. They meet every weekend and go to the cinema. (Natalia)

**1**

**Fostering Socialisation**
- *Build Friendships*
- *Transfer Dramatherapy Experiences at School*

**2**

**Empathy**
- *Understanding Emotions*
- *Stepping in Someone Else's Shoes*

**3**

**Anger and Stress Self-management**
- *Reduction in Tantrums*
- *Enhancing Self-soothing*

**4**

**Acceptance**
- *Hold Space for Others*
- *Being Accepted and Welcomed*

**5**

**Building Bonds within Therapy**
- *Trust Therapists*
- *Connected with Group Members*

**6**

**Promoting Self-expression**
- *Chance to Be Creative*
- *Communicate Feelings and Personal Difficulties*

**7**

**Autonomy**
- *Becoming a Protagonist*
- *Feel Stronger Now*
- *Extending Trust - Not a Little Kid Anymore*

*Figure 9.1* Themes and corresponding subthemes

Also, parents/carers shared that the adolescents' relationships at school have changed in a positive manner as they transferred experiences from the sessions and took initiatives for socialising, e.g., approaching some peers to suggest certain play-drama activities.

He told me he talked to two boys and played together. He told me that one of the boys is really good at telling stories and they play roles just as in the dramatherapy group. (Elias)

The teacher said that she behaves differently at school lately. She suggested that everybody can take up roles and create a theatrical performance. (Stella)

## Empathy

Although every individual thinks and reacts in a unique manner, besides social relationships, parents/carers suggested that they witnessed changes related to the adolescents' skills in identifying and make-meaning of actions and corresponding emotions. In some cases, showing compassion, defending peers and walking a mile in another person's shoes were also reported.

We went to the theatre and he started explaining the actors' emotions during the play, justifying some emotions based on the plot. (Anastasia)

During the last month, I was surprised when he protected bullying victims at school, putting himself in their shoes, saying that they feel 'scared and sad' (Philip).

The adolescents worked with emotions either directly or indirectly during the sessions through stories, improvisations, masks and reflection sharing. Their caregivers reported that some changes in terms of openness, apprehension and controlling emotions promoted trust, connection and spontaneous expression in their family.

Whenever I was telling her 'I love you', she was responding: 'I am not 100% sure what you mean by that but I can only guess that I love you too'. For the first time, she came up to me two weeks ago and said: 'I love you' (Lisa).

Notably, some parents/carers revealed a validation of their observations by an independent professional outside the dramatherapy group.

I discussed that with the child psychiatrist who has been seeing since he was a young child and we agreed that the dramatherapy group has helped him understand circumstances and appropriate emotions. Actually, we now talk way more (Christina).

## Anger and Stress Self-Management

During the interviews, it became clear that adolescents' challenging behaviours or frustration have an emotional impact on caregivers who might feel despondent, especially when the trigger remains unknown. Parents/carers shared examples from their daily life, elaborating on how the absence of tension and edginess can, at times and over time, positively contribute to growth in family bonds and induce parental feelings of hope and optimism. In particular, adolescents' efforts of impulse control and mitigating temper tantrums were discussed.

> The tantrums have been reduced. He stopped yelling 'I hate you'; which happened really often [...]. I cannot express how painful that was. (Anna)
> [...] We even started having conversations about his lack of patience which can be very destructive (Thomas).

Interestingly, adolescents were reported to engage in self-soothing techniques, trying to handle worrying circumstances or stressful thoughts. In fact, the caregivers illustrated how grounding activities employed in the dramatherapy group sessions (i.e., body movement, breathing) were also employed at home.

> It is hard for him to control his compulsions. Lately, I have seen him a couple of times self-soothing, you know. He relaxes his body, lies on the floor, breathing (Christina).
> [...] she was upset and told me she does not want to live in our house anymore [...] asked to spend some time alone [...] she wrote a letter and also, draw a picture for me [...] I think she learned techniques that help her calm down (Lilian).

### Acceptance

The value of acceptance was acknowledged by the caregivers who cherished their adolescents' step-by-step attempts to be somewhat more flexible and stay open to other opinions within the group sessions; witnessing others' views and emotional states as well as offering feedback or giving credit.

> His excessive strictness and rigidness were challenged during all these weeks. I think he learned to hold space for others, without rejecting everyone straight away (Chloe).
> [...] she never changes her mind and wants everybody to agree with her no matter what. In the group, she found her way to listen to others and follow group activities without always being the leader herself (Angel).

At the same time, some parents/carers highlighted their adolescents' motivation driven by feelings of belonging and a sense of recognition that were experienced at the sessions while endorsing the hearty reception in the dramatherapy space by other group members.

He enjoyed being accepted and welcomed in such a warm manner by the others. It was such a gift for us to witness that (Gianna).

He has never got the chance to become a leader of a group activity at school, he is not usually chosen or included by others. He just loved being offered a leading role here, it meant the world to him (Maximus).

### Building Bonds within Therapy

Along with acceptance, almost all parents/carers made explicit references to the emotional bonds that their adolescents created both with the group facilitators and the other group members during the sessions. A strong alliance and trust were confirmed, which in turn motivated the group members to join the sessions while encouraging the more shy or reluctant group members.

At home, she repeats phrases from sessions. She also drew a picture of [the dramatherapist] (Lilian).

We got excited because of his eagerness and joy to come to the sessions without complaining. Frankly, since his early years, he has attended numerous interventions and he is not keen on joining any therapeutic sessions anymore. A couple of times, he asked to call [the dramatherapist] (Alex).

The group cohesiveness was also depicted by parents/carers who made remarks about receiving but also giving peer support in a safe environment. The caregivers shed light on the quality of connection, the sense of community and the corresponding positive influences involving interpersonal learning, shared caring and coping.

He wanted to bring sweets and treats for the group members. He told me that everybody understands him in the group and other children have the same problems in school or at home (Irene).

He told me that during the sessions he talked about things happening in his life and everybody listened to him. I believe this is the reason why he was always calm after sessions (Anna).

### Promoting Self-Expression

According to parents/carers, the safety of the dramatherapy space granted their adolescents the chance to be creative, to express themselves both verbally and nonverbally, and to discover or reveal new talents, skills and preferences. At the same time, some parents believed that creativity and artistic forms within sessions could balance intense school responsibilities, asserting self-expression and positively affecting family communication.

He got the chance to be creative and he is more expressive now. This is evident from the way he describes incidents although he is an introvert. He was proud of the installations and the stories he created (Gianna).

I think that through art, children's hidden talents can be unlocked and expressive abilities are increased. I have read a lot about that. She is so overloaded with school readings and she doesn't often have time to express herself creatively. I am happy for her (Phaedra).

Adolescent self-expression was also warmly appreciated in terms of communicating feelings and personal difficulties in an open and direct way by initiating discussion about their mood state or even disclosing feelings of vulnerability, insecurities and fears.

I couldn't imagine that he carries guilt [...] It helped a lot that he opened about that in the group and maybe he felt that is OK to share that with me as well (Natalia).

He discusses things in life that he wants to change or improve. He told us he would like to speak to a girl, but he does not know how to approach others. He wants to go out more often, but he is scared (Christopher).

### Autonomy

Besides self-expression, during the interviews some caregivers shared their concerns about adaptive behaviour and life skills. They talked about the significance of arts-based activities within a non-judgemental therapeutic space when it comes to interacting in a confident manner and becoming the protagonist instead of avoiding being in the spotlight. Parents/carers realised that their adolescents valued themselves through the eyes of the group members and disclosed that their adolescents' self-worth was enhanced; this, in turn, made a positive contribution in different circumstances of daily life.

He came to me saying that he has a feeling of freedom. He feels free to talk or dance in front of others, he does not feel frightened being the centre of attention (Anastasia).

He managed to become the protagonist instead of just being the spectator in his life. I was so worried about that (Cynthia).

In addition, most caregivers identified and acknowledged their own misconceptions and revealed that they became more open-minded. Through their adolescents' experience of dramatherapy group sessions, parents/carers identified various skills, and behavioural and cognitive aspects of their adolescents' character. The caregivers also realised their low estimation of what their adolescents may be interested in or how they express these interests. They also admitted their own personal shift from viewing the adolescent as a child to handing over responsibility and autonomy.

> At first, we could not believe that our son can be so creative or even talk about his challenges. We are surprised, we had no clue (Zoe).
>
> His behaviour and enthusiasm all throughout these weeks came as a surprise. I don't know, this made me think that maybe we should trust him more (Christina).
>
> He asked to go to the supermarket alone because as he said: 'I am not a little kid any more, I am a grown-up now' (John).

## Discussion

Through 25 qualitative semi-structured interviews, 23 mothers/carers and 16 fathers/carers offered unique observations, insights and recommendations, illuminating changes but also aspects and mechanisms concerning benefits and day-to-day merits of dramatherapy group sessions. Thematic analysis produced seven themes which concerned the benefits of acceptance and bond-building within the dramatherapy group sessions as well as advancements in adolescents' socialisation, empathising abilities, anger and stress self-management, self-expression and autonomy. Most of the present findings agree with previous research studies in this field (e.g., D'Amico et al., 2015; Godfrey and Haythorne, 2013; Tytherleigh and Karkou, 2010; Wilmer-Barbrook, 2013). Similarly, these findings are mostly in line with effects reported by qualified dramatherapists who have shared reflections and vignettes of their clinical experiences through clinical commentaries (e.g., Haythorne and Seymour, 2017; Tricomi and Gallo-Lopez, 2012).

Adolescence has been characterised as a sensitive period entailing major changes in social, emotional and cognitive domains, along with an increasing value of peer relationships. As a result, social skills, perspective-taking and the ability to understand and respond appropriately to others' minds are critical (Valle et al., 2015). According to parents/carers, the adolescents showed increased empathetic behaviour, namely both emotion understanding and appropriate emotion response as well as signs of compassion. Dramatic involvement within the sessions could have facilitated self- and other awareness, through embodiment activities, improvisation and role-playing. At the same time, challenging or maladaptive behaviour is not only one of the main sources of parental anxiety but it may also hinder community integration later in life (Smith and Anderson, 2014). However, working with emotions through different drama activities in the sessions, either in a verbal or nonverbal manner, may have facilitated adolescents' stress reduction, giving them tools to attempt self-regulation and socialisation. This, in turn, promoted connectedness in the family and offered grounds for communication, sharing and adaptation. It has been well-documented that good emotional regulation strategies in children and adolescents with ASD may result in reducing social restraints related to peer relationships while enhancing amusement on social occasions (Goldsmith and Kelley, 2018).

Moreover, the value of acceptance within the dramatherapy sessions was illuminated as this cultivated a sense of belongingness and recognition. According to the parents/carers, some adolescents struggled with growing complexities of social communication, expectations and relationship building at school, thus, experiencing feelings of loneliness or diminished self-worth. Acceptance allowed adolescents to find their own way of self-regulating their perceptions and emotions and respecting other opinions within the group, which might also act as a corrective experience or a disconfirmation of past negative experiences. This is important, as the development of self-esteem can be influenced by emotional understanding, acceptance and feedback from others (McCauley et al., 2019). As well as feeling accepted and accepting others, collaborative bonding and alliance were also reported by the therapists. Literature has shown that the stronger the relationship between therapists and children and adolescents with ASD the better the intervention outcomes are likely to be (Shirk et al., 2011), such as decreasing dysphoria by enhancing positive affect and motivation, and reducing anxiety related to relationship development (Brewe, Mazefsky and White, 2021). Of note, group therapy is a system of many relationships; hence, each member can form an alliance not only with the therapist but also with other members or with the group. The members felt connected either by working towards a common objective (i.e., improvisation, installations, story-making and performance), or by receiving emotional support during sessions. In a similar vein, their self-expression was endorsed by different artistic forms within sessions and they felt safe to share feelings and personal difficulties. Verbalising thoughts and discussing them with others can give a sense of empowerment through self-realisation; this is crucial because adolescents will 'gradually shift their allegiance from home to society and develop an ego identity that is multifaceted but integrated and consistent' (Hanai et al., 2020, p. 1).

Parents/carers also emphasised positive effects on the family, namely hope instillation and optimism, whilst admitting having shifted to trusting their adolescents, acknowledging their capabilities and autonomy. Parents/carers of adolescents with ASD tend to overprotect, they have low expectations for autonomy, and they may intervene whenever a situation becomes challenging (Van Hees et al., 2018). However, allowing adolescents to feel more in control and supporting them to act independently is beneficial for their future. Parental involvement is essential in encouraging adolescents with ASD to build self-determination, choice-making, and risk-taking skills, especially as they enter young adulthood (Hume et al., 2014). Interestingly though, parents/carers recommended the facilitation of dramatherapy group sessions for caregivers to have a supportive space to address their own personal struggles while endorsing their parenting role. Notably, research on arts therapies to support caregivers of children with ASD is scarce, although promising outcomes have been documented when employing dance movement therapy (Aithal et al., 2021).

## Conclusion

Overall, parents/carers perceived that dramatherapy group sessions can support adolescents in different psychosocial domains. Such sessions may also alleviate parental distress and positively impact the family environment. This study engaged a large number of participants who offered their perceptions. They provided a real-life contextual understanding of dramatherapy group sessions for adolescents with ASD, useful for individuals with ASD, their families and practitioners. However, the findings may be culture-bound as all participants came from Western cultures. Also, parents/carers did not mention any adverse effects related to the group sessions. Further research studies could focus on acquiring a sound understanding of how dramatherapy can support not only individuals with ASD across all ages but also their caregivers.

## References

Aithal, S., Karkou, V., Makris, S., Karaminis, T. and Powell, J. (2021) 'Impact of dance movement psychotherapy on the wellbeing of caregivers of children with autism spectrum disorder', *Public Health*, 200, pp. 109–115. Available at: 10.1016/j.puhe.2021.09.018.

American Psychiatric Association. (2013) *Diagnostic and statistical manual of mental disorders, Fifth Edition*. 5th edition. Washington, D.C.: American Psychiatric Publishing.

Bololia, L., Williams, J., Macmahon, K. and Goodall, K. (2022) 'Dramatherapy for children and adolescents with autism spectrum disorder: A systematic integrative review', *Arts in Psychotherapy*, 80(101918). Available at: 10.1016/j.aip.2022.101918.

Brewe, A.M., Mazefsky, C.A. and White, S.W. (2021) 'Therapeutic alliance formation for adolescents and young adults with autism: Relation to treatment outcomes and client characteristics', *Journal of Autism and Developmental Disorders*, 51(5), pp. 1446–1457. Available at: 10.1007/s10803-020-04623-z.

Burrell, T.L. and Borrego, J. (2012) 'Parents' involvement in ASD treatment: What is their role?', *Cognitive and Behavioral Practice*, 19(3), pp. 423–432. Available at: 10.1016/j.cbpra.2011.04.003.

Chesner, A. (1995) *Dramatherapy for people with learning disabilities: A world of difference*. Jessica Kingsley Publishers.

Clarke, V. and Braun, V. (2018) 'Using thematic analysis in counselling and psychotherapy research: A critical reflection', *Counselling and Psychotherapy Research*, 18. Available at: 10.1002/capr.12165.

D'Amico, M., Lalonde, C. and Snow, S. (2015) 'Evaluating the efficacy of drama therapy in teaching social skills to children with autism spectrum disorders', *Drama Therapy Review*, 1(1), pp. 21–40.

Fletcher-Watson, S. and Happé, F. (2019) *Autism: A new introduction to psychological theory and current debate*. 2nd edition. Milton Park, Abingdon, Oxon; New York, NY: Routledge.

Godfrey, E. and Haythorne, D. (2013) 'Benefits of dramatherapy for autism spectrum disorder: A qualitative analysis of feedback from parents and teachers of clients attending roundabout dramatherapy sessions in schools', *Dramatherapy*, 35(1), pp. 20–28. Available at: 10.1080/02630672.2013.773131.

Goldin R.L. and Matson J.L. (2017) 'Current status and future directions', in J.L. Matson (ed.) *Handbook of treatments for autism spectrum disorder*. Springer, pp. 477–484.

Goldsmith, S.F. and Kelley, E. (2018) 'Associations between emotion regulation and social impairment in children and adolescents with autism spectrum disorder', *Journal of Autism and Developmental Disorders*, 48(6), pp. 2164–2173. Available at: 10.1007/s10803-018-3483-3.

Haen, C. and Aronson, S. (2017) *Handbook of child and adolescent group therapy: A practitioner's reference*. New York: Routledge. Available at: 10.4324/9781315 666860.

Hanai, F., Narama, M. and Tamakoshi, K. (2020) 'The self of adolescents with autism spectrum disorder or attention deficit hyperactivity disorder: A qualitative study', *Journal of Autism and Developmental Disorders*, 51(5), pp. 1668–1677. Available at: 10.1007/s10803-020-04653-7.

Haythorne, D. and Seymour, A. (2017) *Dramatherapy and autism*. 1st edition. London; New York: Routledge.

Hume, K., Boyd, B.A., Hamm, J.V. and Kucharczyk, S. (2014) 'Supporting independence in adolescents on the autism spectrum', *Remedial and Special Education*, 35(2), pp. 102–113. Available at: 10.1177/0741932513514617.

Jennings, S. (1999) *Introduction to developmental playtherapy: Playing and health*. Jessica Kingsley Publishers.

Jones, P. (2007) *Drama as therapy Volume 1: Theory, practice and research*. 2nd edn. London: Routledge. Available at: 10.4324/9780203932902.

McCauley, J.B., Harris, M.A., Zajic, M.C., Swain-Lerro, L.E., Oswald, T., McIntyre, N., Trzesniewski, K., Mundy, P. and Solomon, M. (2019) 'Self-esteem, internalizing symptoms, and theory of mind in youth with autism spectrum disorder', *Journal of Clinical Child & Adolescent Psychology*, 48(3), pp. 400–411. Available at: 10.1080/15374416.2017.1381912.

O'Connor, C. and Joffe, H. (2020) 'Intercoder reliability in qualitative research: Debates and practical guidelines', *International Journal of Qualitative Methods*, 19, pp. 1–13.

Onwuegbuzie, A.J. and Leech, N.L. (2007) 'Validity and qualitative research: An oxymoron?', *Quality & Quantity*, 41(2), pp. 233–249. Available at: 10.1007/s11135-006-9000-3.

Reichow, B., Doehring, P., Cicchetti, D.V. and Volkmar, F.R. (eds) (2010) *Evidence-based practices and treatments for children with autism*. 2011th edition. Springer.

Saldaña, J. (2014) 'Coding and Analysis Strategies', in P. Leavy (ed.) *The Oxford handbook of qualitative research*. Oxford University Press. Available at: 10.1093/oxfordhb/9780199811755.013.001.

Shirk, S., Karver, M. and Brown Hangartner, R. (2011) 'The alliance in child and adolescent psychotherapy', *Psychotherapy (Chicago, Ill.)*, 48, pp. 17–24. Available at: 10.1037/a0022181.

Silverman, D. (2005) *Doing Qualitative Research: A Practical Handbook*.SAGE.

Smith, L.E. and Anderson, K.A. (2014) 'The roles and needs of families of adolescents with ASD', *Remedial and Special Education*, 35(2), pp. 114–122. Available at: 10.1177/0741932513514616.

Tricomi, L.P. and Gallo-Lopez, L. (2012) 'The ACT project: Enhancing social competence through drama therapy and performance', in *Play-based interventions for children and adolescents with autism spectrum disorders*. New York, NY, US: Routledge/Taylor & Francis Group, pp. 271–291.

Tytherleigh, L. and Karkou, V. (2010) 'Dramatherapy, autism and relationship-building: A case study', in V. Karkou (ed.) *Arts therapies in schools: Research and practice*. Jessica Kingsley Publishers. pp. 197–216.

Valle, A., Massaro, D., Castelli, I. and Marchetti, A. (2015) 'Theory of mind development in adolescence and early adulthood: The growing complexity of recursive thinking ability', *Europe's Journal of Psychology*, 11(1), pp. 112–124. Available at: 10.5964/ejop.v11i1.829.

Van Hees, V., Roeyers, H. and De Mol, J. (2018) 'Students with autism spectrum disorder and their parents in the transition into higher education: Impact on dynamics in the parent-child relationship', *Journal of Autism and Developmental Disorders*, 48(10), pp. 3296–3310. Available at: 10.1007/s10803-018-3593-y.

Wilmer-Barbrook, C. (2013) 'Adolescence, Asperger's and acting: Can dramatherapy improve social and communication skills for young people with Asperger's syndrome?', *Dramatherapy*, 35(1), pp. 43–56. Available at: 10.1080/02630672.2013.773130.

# Chapter 10

# Looking at the Big Picture

## Caregivers' and Relatives' Life-Worlds on the Contribution of a Combined Dance/Movement and Music Therapy Intervention for Adults with Autism Spectrum Disorder

*Daniel Mateos-Moreno and Lidia Atencia-Doña*

## Introduction

The present study researches an intervention of combined dance/movement and music therapy (DMT and MT) developed by the same authors, which was the object of a published quantitative study in 2013 (Mateos-Moreno and Atencia-Doña). Our aim was to use the combined power of both therapies to explore the benefits for this population. This was challenging in several ways, as it was the first stand-alone, peer-reviewed study investigating an intervention based on the combination of dance/movement therapy (DMT) and music therapy (MT) with adults diagnosed with severe autism. Each session consisted of two halves (an MT and a DMT part), which was challenging in terms of resources and session preparation. Moreover, the activities in the first half-session could affect the second half, e.g., inducing exhaustion in the participants. We tried to compensate for these challenges in uncharted territory by using common sense, e.g., allowing ourselves sufficient on-site preparation time before each session, providing sufficient variety among the activities, using a multisensory approach and developing a dynamic, proactive unfolding of the sessions. The MT half was anchored in the method and musical instruments developed by the German composer and educator Carl Orff (1895-1982), such as beating Orff instruments imitatively and creatively, singing tunes, and corporal percussion. The DMT half was varied, including massaging, simulating situations, imitating or guessing emotions, dancing in different settings, and playing with hoops and balls. These activities adhered to the typical methodology used with ASD individuals in educational contexts, such as errorless learning, shaping, positive and negative reinforcement, and physical restraint (Rivière, 2001; Schmidt, 2004).

In the original study, we researched the impact of the MT and DMT intervention from a quantitative, positivistic paradigm. In the present study, we aim to explore this impact further by capturing the richness of people's experiences guided by a qualitative, interpretivist methodology. Furthermore,

DOI: 10.4324/9781003201656-13

while the previous study had a narrow focus on the in-session behavioural changes of the participants as reported by the Revised Clinical Scale for the Evaluation of Autistic Behaviour (ECA-R) (Barthélémy & Lelord, 2003), we aim in the present study to investigate the consequences of our intervention; including the participants' in-session and off-session behaviours, as well as the life-worlds of their relatives and the caregivers at the participants' care centre. Thus, we aim to investigate the caregivers' and relatives' experiences regarding their impressions, feelings and beliefs about our intervention. The results should, therefore, provide a phenomenological understanding, in the sense of making visible the invisible by searching for the essence of the lived experiences (Merleau-Ponty, 1968).

### Using DMT and MT with ASD Participants

While it is possible to find studies on combined DMT and MT with different client populations (Barnish and Barran, 2020; Dieterich-Hartwell, 2019; Lyons, 2019; Melhuish et al., 2017), to our knowledge, no study other than our original one (Mateos-Moreno and Atencia-Doña, 2013) has been published regarding adults (severely) affected with autism. Moreover, the combination of DMT and MT with autistic children has been reported in a very limited number of studies that evaluate the clients' progression within the intervention. These include the seminal qualitative work of Freundlich, Pike and Schwartz (1989), investigating weekly one-hour sessions of combined DMT and MT carried out in a structured format with autistic children (ranging from 2 to 17 years old; no number of participants or sessions specified). The results of this programme were highly positive from the standpoint of the parents, who reported the following outcomes: increased quality time with their child throughout the interventions, physical exercise for themselves and their children, an opportunity to have fun with their children, chances to share feelings and thoughts with other parents before and after the sessions, and how the children were looking forward to attending the sessions.

Adopting a quantitative methodology, the study pursued by See (2012) included 41 participants (mainly children but one or more adults with age of participants ranging from 2 to 22 years old) who were involved in combined one-hour DMT and MT sessions each week for ten months. The parents who attended the sessions, the music teachers, and some research assistants evaluated the intervention each month by filling a self-designed observational scale (i.e., a Likert scale named the Target Behaviour Checklist, with no data offered on its validation). The findings of this intervention reported an improvement in the participants' scale-defined restlessness (i.e., moving about), fidgeting, temper tantrum, and inattentive behaviours. No significant improvements were found in the scale-defined areas regarding being noisy (shouting or screaming), disruptive behaviours like touching or hitting the others, not following the activities, or freezing up.

Similarly, based on a quantitative methodology, Stamou et al. (2019) researched the impact of 42 thirty-minute sessions based on story-telling, music, and dance on the inclusion of seven autistic children with their typically developing peers in school. The analyses revealed that ASD participants were more engaged with musical activities than with dance or language-focused ones. In addition, a combination of musical and dance activities in the same session fostered the highest levels of physical proximity among participants. By contrast, lower engagement and proximity levels were found for activities solely based on language tasks. Accordingly, the authors concluded that a combination of activities based on music and dance are optimal for promoting the inclusion of ASD children in schools in terms of enhancing their engagement and physical proximity to their peers.

Although it is possible to find a higher number of studies on the independent use of either DMT or MT than those using a combination of these therapies, the research is still limited regarding individuals with ASD. Boso et al. (2007) and Greher et al. (2010) concurrently found that their MT programmes were successful in developing musical skills in adults with ASD. In this case, significant improvements in autism symptoms were observed after six months of starting the MT, with no further improvement at the end of the therapy (i.e., approximately after one year of MT). In addition, Greher et al. (2010) found that MT was motivating and provided benefits in aspects related to social interactions to individuals with ASD.

With respect to the use of DMT with ASD adults, social skills, wellbeing, and an increased awareness of either the self or others is observed across studies (Edwards, 2015; Koch et al., 2015; Koehne et al., 2016). Particularly significant areas of improvement include recognising the needs and emotional states of others (Edwards, 2015; Koehne et al., 2016); improved body awareness (Koch et al., 2015); developing skills for emotional inferences, synchronisation, and imitation (Koehne et al., 2016); and improvement in communicative skills (Wadsworth and Hackett, 2014). However, a more recent study reported no significant changes in the overall empathic levels of the clients from a weekly DMT intervention after 60-minute sessions during a ten-week period (Mastrominico et al., 2018).

In conclusion, the present situation clearly suggests the need for further research on the effects of combining DMT and MT with ASD adults. The gap in the literature is indeed of concern, in view of the aforementioned beneficial effects which have been documented by the separate use of each of these therapies (e.g., Greher et al., 2010; Koehne et al., 2016) and by their combination (Mateos-Moreno and Atencia-Doña, 2013). Furthermore, as several studies have demonstrated (e.g., Freundlich et al., 1989; Melhuish et al., 2017), the perspective of relatives and caregivers may provide important insights to this field of research. In addition, the use of phenomenology has proven well-suited for investigating opinions and impressions in art therapy (Ghetti, 2016) and may thus provide new understandings that cannot be reached through quantitative methodology.

## Study Approach

The clients in our intervention comprised 16 adults (15 males, 1 female) with severe Autistic Spectrum Disorder (ASD) who had scored at least 37 on the Childhood Autism Rating Scale (Schopler et al., 1980). They were divided into two paired groups (control and experimental) of similar ages ($M = 25.31$, $SD = 6.18$). All were inpatients with no previous experience in music or dance at *Centro Pinares* in Malaga (Spain), a care centre led by the non-profit organisation *Autismo Malaga* that did not have any pre-existing programme on Creative Art Therapies (CAT). While the clients continued with their regular activities and pharmacological treatments, those in the experimental group were exposed to 36 one-hour sessions of combined DMT and MT for approximately four and a half months (normally, two sessions per week). For a more detailed description of the intervention, including a sample session, Mateos-Moreno and Atencia-Doña (2013) may be consulted.

The participants in the present study ($n = 6$) pertain to two different groups: the caregivers at the care centre where the intervention was pursued ($n = 5$) and the relatives of the clients with ASD in our intervention ($n = 1$). The inclusion criteria were being present or collaborating at any point during the intervention or having regular contact with any or some of the clients with ASD in the intervention's experimental group. These criteria assured the inclusion of participants capable of appreciating changes in the in-session and off-session behaviours of the clients. The lower number of relatives who accepted our invitation to participate in this study may stem (to some extent) from the fact that they were indirectly recruited through the mediation of the caregivers' group. Moreover, some of the individuals with ASD were full-time residents in the care centre, having only occasional contact with their relatives. However, these facts may not fully account for their families' low response rate; other reasons are unknown to us.

For our approach to research we chose empirical phenomenology, also called transcendental or psychological phenomenology (Moustakas, 1994). This approach allowed us to gain an understanding of the life-worlds of caregivers and relatives around our DMT and MT intervention by suspending our own prejudices (also named *Epoche* or *Bracketing*) 'as much as possible, to take a fresh perspective toward the phenomenon under examination' (Creswell and Poth, 2016, 126). To set aside one's assumptions, it is crucial the one identifies them first (Moustakas, 1994). Following are some statements from our collectively written Epoche that could potentially influence our perspective of the phenomenon:

> We have largely experienced the power of music and dance for the healing and wellbeing of the body and the mind, both in ourselves and in our clients (...) The most powerful outcome that we have experienced

regarding this intervention was the establishment of strong reciprocal links with the clients. Over the course of the interventions, we felt that they were looking forward to meeting us more and more We also felt that we fully succeeded in connecting with them on an emotional level (...) Our perception is that the caregivers were very interested in what we were doing with the clients and always showed appreciation for our work.

The data collection included semi-structured interviews conducted in different moments after terminating the intervention, either in written form (by exchanging several emails, thus allowing for a conversation from both sides) or face-to-face recorded form (approx. one hour each), as well as field diaries and internal reports by the caregivers. Our results were enriched by these multiple methods for collecting data. The interviews were transcribed and aggregated to the rest of the sources, thus compiling a dataset that was subsequently anonymised by substituting the participants' names with alphabetical letters. The primary language used for the data collection was Spanish, and the translations into English were pursued with the aid of a professional language service. The analysis process was undertaken with the help of MaxQDA software. Before and during the analysis, we pursued multiple readings and followed the main steps proposed by Hycner (1999): 1) delineating and refining the units of meaning, 2) building themes by clustering the units of meaning, 3) elaborating summaries, and 4) writing a composite summary, which was the groundwork for the forthcoming results.

## Results

Based on findings from 112 extracts, we will now present the life-worlds of the caregivers and relatives in relation to each of the themes resulting from the analysis.

### General Beliefs on the Content of the Intervention

When the caregivers and relatives commented on the activities, they typically used positive adjectives, such as 'playful' and 'funny'. Furthermore, a common belief in the motivating power of the activities was noted. This power was reported to be associated with music, using expressions such as 'music tends to arouse interest in a high percentage of our group' (I) or 'I have a good opinion on the activities based on the arts as my son is [e] specially motivated by music' (A). Below, a respondent specifies which musical activities were the favourites among the clients with ASD and provides impressions on their performance:

> musical activities: instrumental, sound imitation, body percussion activities, singing, etc. For example, [the activity named] 'Bird', because they

have relaxed in its realisation. They have stretched their arms a lot, and this skill has been more noticeable over the sessions. Everyone wanted to participate with great enthusiasm always in that activity. [The activity named] 'Vocals', where they have taken up the concept of vowels and colour identification. Also, activities related to instruments and songs: They have become better in doing the rhythm and the melody of the songs. They are able to memorise small songs through playing (P).

The same respondent also identified the activities that were less preferred by the adults with ASD, i.e., those containing massages and those where the adults with ASD were lying on the floor.

The respondents identified the development of sensory perception as the most commonly beneficial effect attached to the type of activities that comprised this intervention. In addition, unfolding emotional and communicative skills and the capacity of boosting the power of other therapies were also general beneficial effects attached to CATs by the participants. However, there were two concerns expressed by many respondents regarding these therapies. First, they tend to consider that the effect is highly dependent on individual differences among clients, e.g., 'It is also necessary to bear in mind that it depends on the person. Although music and dance can be motivating for people with ASD, it does not always have to be this way' (I). The other concern pertains to the duration of the therapy: 'These [regarding the therapies] seem adequate to me as long as the intervention based on these therapies is prolonged in time' (M).

### Impact on the Care Centre

The absence of a regular arts therapy programme was the most frequently mentioned aspect regarding how our intervention changed the respondents' life-worlds. Furthermore, they expressed that they have tried to incorporate some of the DMT and MT that they watched in our intervention within their regular activities with ASD patients. Specifically, some respondents argued these activities fostered relaxation and developed imitative skills and sensory perception among the clients with ASD. This fact is fully congruent with the impression that our intervention awoke the caregivers' and relatives' interest in these therapies. Some of the respondents indeed expressed a wish to deepen their knowledge of CAT, even demanding the necessity of in-service training. In addition, one participant declared that, even if they might use what they have learned by watching our intervention, such therapies should be undertaken by trained arttherapists instead of by themselves:

I think that [these types] of activities should be carried out by the right people. I mean those who are trained. It would be good to be trained on this subject [referring to combined DMT and MT] and get to know its benefits. At least for a specific group of clients, as this [the training of the caregivers] would be very good for them (L).

Another respondent expressed that even if there were an attempt to continue with some activities based on CAT beyond our intervention, there were several impediments for doing so:

For a time, it was possible to carry out a series of activities focused on music [after the finalisation of our intervention]; but later, due to the organisation and the functioning of the centre, together with exchanges among centres, we had to suspend those. The activities were mainly related to relaxation and imitation through music (M).

In addition, positive attitudes towards the therapists were also developed by the respondents, e.g.:

The sensitivity, commitment, and collaboration that you show with your contribution encourage us [referring to the caregivers at the care centre] to continue working and enable people affected by this serious disability to benefit from a much-needed project, helping to improve their quality of life (J).

### The Clients' Off-Session Behaviours

The most common effect observed among clients outside the intervention was an improvement in their communicative skills. Most often mentioned were an enrichment of the individuals' vocabulary and and increase in their communicative attempts. The following answer epitomises many others:

With regard to language, certain users are not able to execute vowel emissions. There has been no improvement on that, but [I saw] an increased intention on their part with gazes and noises. In terms of those who are capable of speaking, I observed that they have enriched their language (P).

Likewise, a common aspect highlighted by the respondents regards how individuals with ASD developed a high motivation for attending the sessions. This is relevant, as one respondent explained, 'given the difficulty of adults with ASD to widen their interests' (I).

Other positive outcomes highlighted by some respondents include their perception of an improvement in the clients' quality of life, happiness, and daily satisfaction. These effects were perceived mainly before and after each session. In addition, some respondents noticed how the adults with ASD established an emotional link with the therapists, e.g., 'On some occasions, they asked us about Lidia, [asking] for example: When is Lidia coming?' (P). In addition, some perceived outcomes related to musical abilities: developing musical skills and showing an increased reaction or sensibility to music. This was appreciated by how the adults with ASD moved and produced vocal utterances spontaneously when they listened to music. One of the respondents' expressions is specific in terms of what musical skills were perceived as improved: 'They have improved [doing] the rhythm and the melody of songs. They are [now] able to memorise small songs' (P). This respondent explains that the adults with ASD also repeated the movements and songs practiced in the sessions in other contexts outside of the intervention with or without music. These perceived positive effects contrast with impressions of how some of the typical autistic behaviours remained unaffected outside of the intervention, mostly regarded as the ability for social interactions and stereotyped behaviours. In addition, the respondents expressed that they observed no long-term benefit after the intervention was concluded. Moreover, two respondents reflect on how difficult it is to do unstructured, qualitative assessments with individuals experiencing severe ASD:

> It is difficult to assess any changes of these individuals due to the severity of their conditions. Furthermore, many times they tend to have regressive changes or associated mental disorders, such as depressive disorders or melancholy, which are not caused by environmental factors but by endogenous ones derived from their pathologies, which tends to aggravate it [i.e., the difficulties in assessing off-session behaviours] (I)

### The In-Session Behaviours of Adults with ASD

The most commonly referred to positive outcome observed within the sessions was what the respondents term the clients' 'initiative', understood as the clients' intention to join in the activities and sustain their engagement. This outcome, as some respondents explained, was progressively achieved throughout multiple sessions. Additional positive outcomes highlighted by the respondents include their perceptions of the clients' 'satisfaction' and how they were perceived as feeling 'less isolated'. Improvements in specific domains, such as empathy and imitative abilities and the ability to pay attention or concentrate on something, were also mentioned by many respondents. The following answer exemplifies how some of these aspects were explained:

> With regard to the neurophysiological function, the user had the most positive results in [the ability of] imitation, showing at moments no great difficulty in mimicking movements or sounds, as well as imitating the emotions expressed by others (P).

Some respondents observed the adults with ASD being more relaxed, with less stereotyped behaviours and better control of their motor skills during the sessions. However, the stereotyped behaviours never fully disappeared during the sessions, as recalled by one respondent. This respondent also highlighted that some adults showed frustration or restlessness at some points but attributes the behaviours to endogenous factors as these were common off-session behaviours, too.

The clients are commonly regarded to have shown an increased awareness of their bodies during the sessions, with no signs of rejection towards the activities and having generally fewer symptoms of ASD behaviours. The clients' capacity to establish social interactions is also believed to have increased during the sessions.

## Discussion

Unlike typical studies on CAT with autistic clients (e.g., Boso et al., 2007; Edwards, 2015; See, 2012), we were successful in addressing the experienced impact of art-based interventions outside of the interventions' framework, i.e., investigating how the adults with ASD are seen to feel and behave in other contexts. Moreover, we have explored the impact of the intervention in the life-worlds of the caregivers and relatives of individuals with ASD. The most relevant global result, then, is that the lived experiences of the participants in this study showed no negative effect from these therapies. Instead, there are many positive outcomes that would justify the inclusion of regular combined DMT and MT with the client group concerned in this case.

Our results are fully coincident with those in previous studies (Freundlich, Pike and Schwartz, 1989; Greher et al., 2010) in identifying the clients' high motivation to participate in CAT. Furthermore, the clients in our study are described as happier, with higher daily satisfaction and a better quality of life in their regular activities outside the intervention. These effects are more noticeable before and after each session, which supports the existence of a causal relation. Off-session positive effects also included improvements in the clients' communicative skills, namely an enriched vocabulary and increased communicative attempts, developing musical skills and sensitivity to music, and establishing emotional links with the therapists.

Regarding the behaviours of adults with ASD during the sessions, their self-initiative to undertake a task is the most commonly mentioned positive effect as observed by the caregivers and relatives. In addition, there are many varied positive effects described by one or more of the participants in this study: an impression of the adults with ASD feeling less isolated and displaying increased empathic levels, improved imitative skills, better attention/concentration, greater relaxation, fewer stereotyped behaviours, finer control of motor skills, better body awareness, and an increased capacity to establish social interactions. While many of these outcomes are fully supported by the quantitative results of our previous study, others are difficult to relate to the dimensions captured by the ECA-R scale that we used to track clients' evolution (Mateos-Moreno & Atencia-Doña, 2013). With respect to these concordances, all of the aspects positively affected as measured by the ECA-R

scale are compatible with those found in the lived experiences of the participants in this study, such as better self-regulation, increased empathic abilities,
and being less fidgety. Furthermore, these positive outcomes are also fully
coincident with the results of previous studies on CAT (Edwards, 2015;
Koehne et al., 2016; See, 2012). However, an exception may be found in the
study of Mastrominico et al. (2018), which found that the empathic levels of
adults with ASD remained unchanged even after DMT. We hypothesise that a
possible explanation for this discrepancy may be that a combination of MT
and DMT gave better results than using these therapies independently.
Moreover, the respondents in our study consistently attached the motivation
to engage in the therapy to the activities related to music, in alignment with the
results of Stamou et al. (2019) comparing the engagement in musical activities
versus dance/movement activities among adults with ASD.

In terms of the discordances between the present study and our previous
one (Mateos-Moreno & Atencia-Doña, 2013) on the impact of the intervention, the most shocking aspect regards the ECA-R function defined as 'intention', which may be paralleled by what the participants at the present study
name the clients' *initiative*: while this aspect was not found to change significantly in the previous study, all the participants in the present study deemed
the clients' initiative as improved during the sessions. This inconsistency may
lie in the variable operationalisation, as the ECA-R defined function of
'intention' refers to multiple aspects (e.g., agitation, restlessness, compulsive-
ness) in addition to the clients' self-initiative to engage in the activities. This
may indicate a need for a revision of this dimension in the scale.

In comparing the clients' in-session and off-session behaviours, there is a
clear discrepancy in two aspects: 1) Typical ASD-stereotyped behaviours
were perceived to decrease during the sessions, though they were perceived
to be unchanged outside the sessions; 2) Social abilities were regarded as
increased during the sessions and simultaneously unchanged in other contexts. Given the limited duration of our intervention, we hypothesise that a
longer-term intervention combining DMT and MT might help in the transfer
of the beneficial effects of these therapies to off-session contexts.

A remarkable result is how our intervention positively influenced not only
the individuals with ASD (as concurrently found by the present and previous
study on this intervention) but also the life-worlds of the caregivers and the
relatives involved in the present study. For example, after the intervention
was finished, the caregivers tried, with more or less success, to incorporate
within their regular work with these individuals some of the activities that
they saw in our intervention. Furthermore, the participants in our study
deemed their lack of knowledge of these therapies as a weakness and
reflected on the necessity of recruiting accredited therapists on CAT for
developing these therapies at the care centre. However, CAT was always
conceived as a complement to other therapies, and its effect was seen as
dependent on both the individual differences of the clients and the duration

of the therapies. In addition, no long-lasting effect was appreciated after the completion of our intervention, which suggests that such an intervention might only have an impact either during its length or if developed for a longer period of time.

## Conclusion

This study provides solid evidence for the positive lived experiences of the participants and thus supports exploring the incorporation of a combination of MT and DMT within the regular activities of adults with severe ASD. However, like all case studies, it is impossible to draw generalisations further than those of a naturalistic character, i.e., generalisations done by the reader and based on the similarities among the contexts and the specific participants (Stake, 1995). In addition, further studies including more participants could provide better data saturation and may reveal aspects not found in our analysis. Future research may also replicate the use of mixed methodologies in exploring similar interventions to contrast our results. Finally, the investigation of the off-session behaviour of individuals with ASD and the lifeworlds of the others (e.g., relatives and caregivers) on CAT has been unveiled as an area in need of further research for supporting or contradicting the results found in the present study.

## References

Barnish, M.S. and Barran, S.M. (2020) 'A systematic review of active group-based dance, singing, music therapy and theatrical interventions for quality of life, functional communication, speech, motor function and cognitive status in people with Parkinson's disease', *BMC Neurology*, 20, p. 371. Available at: 10.1186/s12 883-020-01938-3.

Barthélémy, C. and Lelord, G. (2003) *Échelle d_Évaluation des Comportements Autistiques. Manuel ECAR-T (Version Revise).* [Scale for the Evaluation of Autistic Behavior. Handbook for the ECAR-T (Revised Version)]. Editions et Applications Psychologiques (EAP).

Boso, M., Emanuele, E., Minazzi, V., Abbamonte, M. and Politi, P. (2007) 'Effect of long-term interactive music therapy on behavior profile and musical skills in young adults with severe autism', *The Journal of Alternative and Complementary Medicine*, 13(7), pp. 709–712. Available at: 10.1089/acm.2006.6334.

Creswell, J.W. and Poth, C.N. (2016) *Qualitative inquiry and research design: Choosing among five approaches*. SAGE Publications.

Dieterich-Hartwell, R.M. (2019) 'Music, movement, and emotions: an inquiry with suggestions for the practice of dance/movement therapy', *Body, Movement and Dance in Psychotherapy*, 14(4), pp. 249–263. Available at: 10.1080/17432979. 2019.1676310.

Edwards, J. (2015) 'Exploring sensory sensitivities and relationships during group dance movement psychotherapy for adults with autism', *Body, Movement and Dance in Psychotherapy*, 10(1), pp. 5–20. Available at: 10.1080/17432979.2014.978894.

Freundlich, B.M., Pike, L.M. and Schwartz, V. (1989) 'Dance and music for children with autism', *Journal of Physical Education, Recreation & Dance*, 60(9), pp. 50–53. Available at: 10.1080/07303084.1989.10609812.

Ghetti, C.M. (2016) 'Phenomenological research in music therapy', in J. Edwards (ed.) *The Oxford handbook of music therapy*. Oxford University Press, Available at: 10.1093/oxfordhb/9780199639755.013.15.

Greher, G.R., Hillier, A., Dougherty, M. and Poto, N. (2010) 'SoundScape: An interdisciplinary music intervention for adolescents and young adults on the autism spectrum', *International Journal of Education & the Arts*, 11(9). Available at: https://www.learntechlib.org/p/52009/ (Accessed 28 August 2022).

Koch, S.C., Mehl, L., Sobanski, E., Sieber, M. and Fuchs, T. (2015) 'Fixing the mirrors: A feasibility study of the effects of dance movement therapy on young adults with autism spectrum disorder', *Autism: The International Journal of Research and Practice*, 19(3), pp. 338–350. Available at: 10.1177/1362361314522353.

Koehne, S., Behrends, A., Fairhurst, M.T. and Dziobek, I. (2016) 'Fostering social cognition through an imitation- and synchronization-based dance/movement intervention in adults with autism spectrum disorder: A controlled proof-of-concept study', *Psychotherapy and Psychosomatics*, 85(1), pp. 27–35. Available at: 10.1159/000441111.

Lyons, S. (2019) *Arts therapies for dementia: a systematic review and community-based case study on the value of music therapy and dance movement therapy*. PhD. Edge Hill University.

Mastrominico, A., Fuchs, T., Manders, E., Steffinger, L., Hirjak, D., Sieber, M., Thomas, E., Holzinger, A., Konrad, A., Bopp, N. and Koch, S.C. (2018) 'Effects of dance movement therapy on adult patients with autism spectrum disorder: A randomized controlled trial', *Behavioral Sciences (Basel, Switzerland)*, 8(7), p. E61. Available at: 10.3390/bs8070061.

Mateos-Moreno, D. and Atencia-Doña, L. (2013) 'Effect of a combined dance/movement and music therapy on young adults diagnosed with severe autism', *The Arts in Psychotherapy*, 40(5), pp. 465–472. Available at: 10.1016/j.aip.2013.09.004.

Melhuish, R., Beuzeboc, C. and Guzmán, A. (2017) 'Developing relationships between care staff and people with dementia through music therapy and dance movement therapy: A preliminary phenomenological study', *Dementia (London, England)*, 16(3), pp. 282–296. Available at: 10.1177/1471301215588030.

Merleau-Ponty, M. (1968) *The visible and the invisible (studies in phenomenology and existential philosophy)*. 1st edition. Evanston, Ill: Northwestern University Press.

Moustakas, C. (1994) *Phenomenological research methods*. 1st edition. Thousand Oaks, Calif: SAGE Publications, Inc.

Rivière, Á. (2001) *Autismo: Orientaciones para la intervención educativa*. 1st edition. Madrid: Editorial Trotta, S.A.

Schmidt, B.H. (2004) *Autism in the school-aged child: Expanding behavioral strategies and promoting success by Beth Heybyrne*. Autism Family Press.

Schopler, E., Reichler, R.J., DeVellis, R.F. and Daly, K. (1980) 'Toward objective classification of childhood autism: Childhood Autism Rating Scale (CARS)', *Journal of Autism and Developmental Disorders*, 10(1), pp. 91–103. Available at: 10.1007/BF02408436.

See, C.M. (2012) 'The use of music and movement therapy to modify behaviour of children with autism', *Pertanika Journal of Social Science and Humanities*, 20, pp. 1103–1116.

Stake, R.E. (1995) *The art of case study research*. Thousand Oaks: Sage Publications. Available at: http://books.google.com/books?id=sIMOAQAAMAAJ (Accessed 28 August 2022).

Stamou, A., Bonneville-Roussy, A., Ockelford, A. and Terzi, L. (2019) 'The effectiveness of a music and dance program on the task engagement and inclusion of young pupils on the autism spectrum', *Music & Science*, 2, pp. 1–12. Available at: 10.1177/2059204319881852.

Wadsworth, J. and Hackett, S. (2014) 'Dance movement psychotherapy with an adult with autistic spectrum disorder: An observational single-case study', *Body, Movement and Dance in Psychotherapy*, 9(2), pp. 59–73. Available at: 10.1080/17432979.2014.893259.

# Part III

# Coming Together with Hatchlings – Arts Therapies in Different Combinations and Conditions

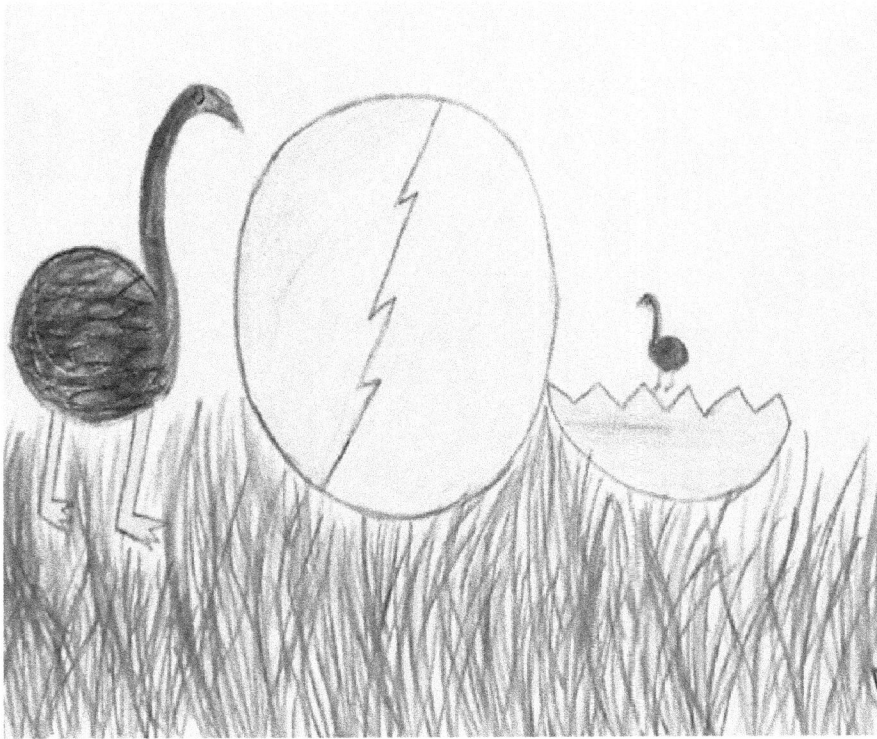

# Chapter 11

# Adapting to COVID-19

## Tele-Dance Movement Psychotherapy for Children and Adolescents with Autism

*Janet Tein Ni Moo and Rainbow Tin Hung Ho*

## Introduction

### Social Distancing During COVID-19 and Suspended Services

In the climate caused by the COVID-19 pandemic, meeting up physically posed health risks whilst social distancing was difficult to maintain when meeting with children who were used to certain levels of physical interaction. Consequently, schools around the world had to close fully or partially. According to UNESCO, on 24th April 2020, a high percentage of 84.5% of the total amount of enrolled learners globally (at pre-primary, primary, secondary, and tertiary education levels) were impacted by school closures, with 166 country-wide closures. Typically, schools do not merely provide education but, amongst other things, they also provide a sense of routine and structure, physical activity, opportunities for social interaction, and therapeutic activities. School closures, coupled with the suspension of services such as intervention centres, resulted in children and adolescents losing important resources, possibly hampering their development and affecting their wellbeing.

Although schools did adapt to the coronavirus, many were still closed intermittently, offering limited services and functioning within the coronavirus restrictions. Additionally, the cycles of starting back at school and then pausing in response to rising COVID-19 cases led to a need to transition back and forth between school and home.

### The Impact of COVID-19: Disruptions to Children and Adolescents with ASD

For individuals with Autism Spectrum Disorder (ASD) in particular, such disruptions to their routine and the need to constantly adapt around the COVID-19 restrictions and home confinement have been especially distressing. These disruptions may have had a particularly strong impact on children and adolescents with ASD who have psychiatric vulnerabilities and comorbidities (American Psychiatric Association, 2013). In a meta-analysis

DOI: 10.4324/9781003201656-15

investigating co-occurring mental health diagnoses in autism (Lai et al., 2019), the respective pooled estimates were, for example, 28% for Attention Deficit Hyperactivity Disorder, 20% for anxiety, 11% for depression, and 9% for obsessive compulsive disorder. As noted by Ameis and her colleagues (2020), the pandemic was expected to particularly impact individuals with ASD with more behavioural difficulties, who, prior to COVID-19, had experienced sleep and attention dysregulation, anxiety, depressive symptoms, and those who are on psychotropic medication.

The detrimental impact on children with ASD and their families was reported in the news from the early stages of the pandemic, for example, in Hong Kong, where residential space constraints may have worsened matters. Citing families of children with ASD, a report from Hong Kong (Sun, 2020) described how disrupted routines, ensuing emotional problems, and being trapped at home led to conflicts with parents and self-inflicted injuries. Consistent with such news reports, Ameis and colleagues (2020) listed possible effects, such as exacerbation of problematic restricted and repetitive behaviours, sleep problems, and aggression, commonly directed towards caregivers. All these undoubtedly led to increased parental stress.

Online learning and being at home may have benefited some children and adolescents with ASD who are more comfortable in their home environment, with a self-paced schedule, and opportunities to engage in self-soothing behaviours without adverse social implications (Ameis et al., 2020). Furthermore, a recent survey in the UK (Pavlopoulou et al., 2020) involving 449 participants found that 70% of family carers of children or young persons with ASD reported that their daily routines changed because of COVID-19; interestingly, many of them preferred not to return to their world pre-COVID. This research outcome may indicate a need for a shift in care delivery.

In summary, although certain shifts in the routines of individuals with ASD and their families have been welcome and may lead to changes in the future, the disruptions brought on by COVID-19 might have been stressful in general. As such, for those children with ASD who were previously engaged with psychotherapy, there may have been a need to continue psychotherapy online (Narzisi, 2020). It is also important to consider the use of technology as means to make provision accessible and flexible not only as a response to the crisis as it evolved (Ameis et al., 2020), but also post-crisis.

### Tele-Dance Movement Psychotherapy with Children and Adolescents with ASD

Dance Movement Psychotherapy (DMP) has been reported to be beneficial for individuals with ASD. DMP refers to a relational process in which body movement and dance are used as instruments of communication during the psychotherapeutic process (Association of Dance Movement Psychotherapy UK, 2013). Due to DMP's focus on body movement as an instrument of communication and expression, it has a unique role in working with individuals with ASD, given their atypical social communication. In a systematic review (Takahashi et al., 2019) of the effectiveness of DMP interventions in autism, it was found that mirroring interventions and their variations helped enhance the social skills of individuals with ASD.

In terms of children with ASD, the benefits of DMP are highlighted in Scharoun's (2014) narrative review in which she concluded that DMP can be beneficial, both physically and psychologically. A recent systematic review (Aithal et al., 2021a) on this topic suggested that DMP can potentially promote wellbeing in several ways but as it stands, the evidence for its effectiveness is inconclusive due to the quality of available studies. An independent review of available literature revealed that positive outcomes include improvements in the social and communication domains (Aithal et al., 2021b; Baudino, 2010; Partelli, 1995; Samaritter and Payne, 2017); changes in patterns or behaviours (Partelli, 1995); improvements in regulatory behaviour and influence on the sensory systems (Devereaux, 2017); and fewer incidents of violent outbursts (Torrance, 2003).

During the COVID-19 pandemic, it was difficult to facilitate DMP services in person, as interacting physically posed health risks and social distancing was difficult to maintain when meeting with children with Special Educational Needs and Disabilities (SEND). One solution was teletherapy. Although there was no literature on tele-DMP and autism, a systematic review (Sutherland et al., 2018) examining a range of telehealth services and autism at the time of this study, including diagnostic assessments, early intervention, and language therapy, had suggested that children with autism, their families, and teachers may benefit from using telehealth. This served as a prelude to the usefulness of tele-DMP in autism.

Since then, a study on family-centred tele-DMP with children with autism has found both benefits and challenges (Moo & Ho, 2023). Positive outcomes include the child's social development; enjoyment; parents' improved understanding of the child; insight and ideas; and relationship building, whilst difficulties included screen-to-screen interactions; home; and physical distance (Moo & Ho, 2023).

### Objectives

This study aimed to investigate the use of tele-DMP for children and adolescents with ASD during the current COVID-19 pandemic in Hong Kong (HK), the United Kingdom (UK), Australia, and New Zealand.

## Study Approach

### Recruitment

This study obtained ethical approval from the Human Research Ethics Committee of the University of Hong Kong. Following that, Hong Kong-, UK-,

Australia-, and New Zealand-based dance movement therapists working with children or adolescents with ASD using teletherapy were recruited via personal contacts of the authors and emails sent out by the relevant professional organisations of DMP in each region, namely the Hong Kong Dance Movement Therapy Association (HKDMTA), the Association of Dance Movement Psychotherapy UK (ADMP UK), and the Dance Therapy Association of Australasia (DTAA).

### Procedure

After giving their consent, the recruited dance movement therapists took part in interviews online via Zoom with one of the authors (both authors are dance movement therapists). The semi-structured interviews in English focused on three topics, namely (i) therapeutic elements or methods present in their tele-DMP; (ii) outcomes; and (iii) concerns and considerations in using tele-DMP. Their recorded interviews were then transcribed and analysed. Discussions were held between the two authors when there were discrepancies in data interpretation until a consensus was reached.

### Qualitative Data Analyses

The interview texts were analysed using Thematic Network Analysis (Attride-Stirling, 2001), a method of organising thematic analysis of qualitative data, sitting within a constructivist school of thought. Constructivism maintains that there is no objective reality, and researchers are always actively involved in constructing their own knowledge. This subjective reality is reached by linking new information and experiences with prior learning. This paradigm was helpful as both authors are dance movement therapists who have worked with children and adolescents with ASD and it engaged their prior experience to inform interpretation of the texts.

In this study, the rich data supplied by the four participants shared underlying themes but also differences. Hence, thematic network analysis was helpful to structure this. Following the procedures of thematic network analysis, texts were first scanned for codes using a coding framework devised by the author (Braun and Clarke, 2006). The coding framework was based on the three main questions asked during the interview. Each of those three topics generated codes and for each code, the issues discussed were listed, forming the basic themes.

The basic themes were then clustered into the organising themes, and from there, interpreted to arrive at the global themes. These are 'superordinate themes that encompass the principal metaphors in the data as a whole' (Attride-Stirling, 2001, p. 5). A distinctive feature of this method of analysis is the 'web-like network', which is not the analysis itself. Rather, it is used as 'an organising principle and illustrative tool' (Attride-Stirling, 2001, p. 4) for analysis, which requires interpretation of the text. To enhance the trustworthiness of the study, the second author, who is the academic supervisor of the first author, reviewed the analyses of the first author. Any discrepancies in opinion were resolved through discussion between the two authors to reach a consensus.

## Results

Four dance movement therapists (DS, K, T, and R, identified in full in the acknowledgements section) responded to the invitation to take part in this study, with two from the United Kingdom, one from Hong Kong, and one based in New Zealand. They comprised three females and one male and had an average age of 46 years. Their mean years of working experience as a dance movement therapist in general and with children and adolescents with ASD were respectively 11.4 years and 9.5 years. The interviews lasted from 30 to 60 minutes each. Using Thematic Network Analysis as described in the methods section above, the transcriptions of their interviews were analysed.

The first topic, 'Therapeutic elements or methods', generated 20 codes, the second topic, 'Outcomes' generated 3 codes, and the third topic, 'Concerns and considerations' generated 5 codes. For each code, the issues discussed were listed, and these issues formed the basic themes. Table 11.1 illustrates this with three example codes for each topic.

All the basic themes were then clustered into organising themes, which were in turn, interpreted into global themes. Table 11.2 illustrates this with one example for each topic.

In terms of organising themes, for 'Therapeutic elements or methods', the themes were 'Mirroring and attuning', 'Meeting them where they are', 'Playing', 'Using structure', 'Holding', 'Music', 'Using devices to facilitate audio-visual perception that is more like real life', 'Utilising space in 2D to convey space in reality', 'Using aids to visualise externally', 'Using verbal and vocal means', 'Moving freely, more like real life', 'Using devices to reduce the frame', 'Working with smaller movements', and 'Having an internal anchor for movement'.

In terms of 'Outcomes', the organising themes were 'Positive feelings', 'Connecting with others', 'Different reactions to the screen, resulting in varying attendance rates', 'Internal self-reflection', 'Maintenance of well-being', 'Creativity and new possibilities for clients', 'New perspectives for parents', and 'Therapist development'.

The organising themes for 'Concerns and considerations in using tele-therapy' were 'Lack of bodily cues', 'Essentiality of physical contact', 'Difficulty in building the therapeutic relationship', 'Limitations of using the screen', 'Time to plan creatively', and 'Difficulty involving parents'.

All the organising themes were then interpreted to reach the global themes. Table 11.2 illustrates the interpreting from organising themes to global themes, with one example from each topic. For 'Therapeutic methods or elements', these global themes were 'Tele-DMP as therapy as

Table 11.1 From codes to themes

| Codes (Step 1) | Issues discussed | Themes identified (Step 2) |
|---|---|---|
| | **Therapeutic elements or methods** | |
| Movement | • Movement as cues<br>• Size of movement<br>• Facial expressions<br>• Movement practices<br>• Types of movement<br>• Sitting<br>• Internal focus<br>• Previous movement experience with therapist<br>• Body language<br>• Therapist's freedom to move | • Utilising space in camera to explore polarities (DS,K), e.g., in and out, big and small, front and back<br>• Little movements are important too (DS)<br>• Responding to clients' small and distinctive movements and gestures (DS)<br>• If you can, observe their movements and reflect (K)<br>• Interesting micromovements in facial expressions, e.g., 'happy face' - clients are more focused and willing to engage as they like electronic things such as the camera and feel safer (K)<br>• Mindfulness movement (K)<br>• Rhythmic movement (K)<br>• Not necessarily big movements (K)<br>• Very much sitting in a chair and containing (R)<br>• At most, breathing, body scan, and grounding in a chair, if clients are in the right environment (R)<br>• More internal, meditative, and explorative work (T)<br>• Would only explore how we move through space in 2D with clients who have already done movement together with therapist before in real life (T)<br>• In teletherapy, the scene is set verbally; movements are more in terms of body language (T)<br>• Telephone therapy gives the therapist freedom to move (T) |
| Space in camera | • Polarities<br>• Reality<br>• Sense of moving<br>• Distance | • Utilising space in camera to explore polarities (DS,K), e.g., in and out, big and small, front and back<br>• Using space to remind clients that therapists are real as reality becomes less distinct in 2D, thus letting clients see the space and have a sense of moving and crossing distance (T) |
| Holding | • Safe holding space<br>• Different platforms<br>• Managing anxiety<br>• Being with difficulties | • Being mindful and letting clients feel safe first, with a 'less is more' approach (K)<br>• Recognising integral knowledge in holding the group and holding the individual, even on the screen-to-screen platform (R)<br>• Creating safe holding space (R)<br>• Managing anxiety (R)<br>• Being with as best we can and not running away from problems or difficult feelings (T) |

(Continued)

*Table 11.1* (Continued)

| Codes (Step 1) | Issues discussed | Themes identified (Step 2) |
|---|---|---|
| | | **Outcomes** |
| *Benefits to clients* | • Positive feelings<br>• Connection<br>• Creativity<br>• Parents' perception<br>• Different reactions to the screen<br>• Varying attendance rates<br>• Security<br>• Internal self-reflection<br>• Maintenance | • Adolescents verbalised that they were happy after taking part in sound and movement and imagery exercises (K)<br>• Children were happy to jump around during a time when they had been stuck at home because of the pandemic (K)<br>• Children felt happy and playful following activities utilising space in the camera to explore polarities (K)<br>• The children felt seen in the give and take and sharing of movements (DS)<br>• Each member was acknowledged, and a sense of connection, support and wellness was fostered through repetitive common movements (DS)<br>• Using household items as props opened creativity (DS)<br>• Parents learned to appreciate little movements (DS)<br>• New attendees benefited from the layer of security offered by the screen (R)<br>• Clients dropped in number but those who attended did so religiously (R)<br>• Clients' explored internal self-reflection, especially with telephone therapy which is more defined whilst more remote (T)<br>• Maintenance: Clients who did teletherapy were in a better place and less withdrawn than those who stopped therapy altogether (T) |
| *Neutral observations* | • Altered group dynamics | • Children observed the therapist more than other children (K) |
| *Therapist development* | • New perspective<br>• Enriched practice<br>• Skill set<br>• Inventive and creative | • At first, the therapist was against using Zoom, thinking 'How will it work?' as the most important thing to her is body contact, ('We will lose everything') but now having done teletherapy, the therapist realises that remaining at home can feel like a safe place for children and parents, and sessions can even be more focused (DS)<br>• Screen-to-screen is a platform that the therapist would never have considered if she had not been forced into it because of the global pandemic. However, it has actually enriched her practice and added to her skillset (R)<br>• The therapist saw new possibilities and became more inventive and creative (T) |

(Continued)

*Table 11.1* (Continued)

| Codes (Step 1) | Issues discussed | Themes identified (Step 2) |
|---|---|---|
| **Concerns and considerations** | | |
| *Bodily cues* | • Lack of bodily feedback<br>• Lack of kinaes-thetic empathy<br>• Lack of bodily cues<br>• Contrast to real life | • There is a lack of immediate bodily feedback from the children, e.g., holding hands (K)<br>• Certain techniques may be less suitable in teletherapy, such as Authentic Movement, as there is less kinaesthetic empathy compared to real life (K)<br>• Prefers being together in the room for its richness in terms of being able to pick up bodily cues, as it is mentally exhausting trying to pick up cues that are not visible on screen (R)<br>• In real life, we would have movement - inter-actional shaping, rhythm, and flow - as sources of information (T) |
| *Physical contact* | • Passing and sharing of props<br>• Physical being with<br>• Essential to human life<br>• View of the body in a pandemic<br>• Responsibility as dance movement therapists<br>• Therapeutic rela-tionship<br>• Avoidant client | • Depth of work is lost without the passing and sharing of props physically (R)<br>• The therapist hardly does online work now as he deeply values physically being with in person, face-to-face (T)<br>• Caution against keeping therapy online as physical contact is essential to human life and screen-to-screen can be deeply alienating and lonely (T)<br>• During this pandemic when bodies are seen as contaminating, it is our responsibility as dance movement therapists to 'put ourselves in the danger zone' since therapists should not run away from problems, but be with them as best we can, in the circumstances (T)<br>• Teletherapy can be an introduction to the internal world of children with ASD, albeit a chaotic one, but can be hopeless in terms of the therapeutic relationship, if the child is avoidant or hyperactive (T) |
| *Parents* | • Sacrifice time<br>• See children with different eyes | • May be unready to sacrifice their time (DS)<br>• May be uncomfortable to take a step back to listen to their children and see them with different eyes as it is a big step to see every little thing as significant (DS) |

usual', 'Tele-DMP as a window', and 'Tele-DMP as a filter'. For 'Outcomes', these were 'Positive feelings', 'Maintenance', and 'New possibilities and developments'. For 'Concerns and considerations', these were 'Importance of physical interactions', 'The therapeutic space', and 'Future work'. Table A in the Appendix lists all the basic, organising, and global themes.

Table 11.2 From basic themes to global themes

| Basic themes | Organising themes | Global themes |
| --- | --- | --- |
| **Therapeutic methods or elements** | | |
| Responding to clients' small and distinctive movements and gestures (DS) | Working with smaller movements | Teletherapy as a filter |
| Managing parents' expectations by reminding them that little movements are important too (DS) | Having an internal anchor for movement, e.g., mindfulness, internal reflections, previous experience of moving together with a therapist, verbal checking and understanding, sitting | |
| Interesting micromovements in facial expressions, with clients more focused and willing to engage as they like electronic things like the camera and feel safer (K) | | |
| Not necessarily big movements (K) | | |
| Mindfulness movement (K) | | |
| Very much sitting in a chair and containing (R) | | |
| At most, breathing, body scan, and grounding in a chair, if clients are in the right environment (R) | | |
| More internal, meditative, and explorative work (T) | | |
| Would only explore how we move through space in 2D with clients who have already done movement together with the therapist before (T) | Using devices to reduce the frame | |
| In teletherapy, the scene is set verbally, movement is more in terms of body language (T) | | |
| Verbal checking and understanding (T) | | |
| Using telephone therapy, which is more defined but more remote, like text (T) | | |
| Clients hiding self-view in telephone therapy reduces the frame, encourages internal self-reflection, and is more like real life (T) | | |
| Voice is intimate and encourages internal self-reflection, in telephone therapy (T) | | |
| **Outcomes** | | |
| Clients explored internal self-reflection, especially with telephone therapy which is more defined whilst more remote (T) | Internal self-reflection | New possibilities and development |
| Individuals who had previously never engaged in therapy available to them began attending sessions (R) | New attendees | |
| Using household items as props opened creativity (DS) | Creativity | |
| It enabled clients to see new possibilities (T) | New perspectives for parents | |
| Parents learned to appreciate little movements (DS) | Therapist development | |

(Continued)

Table 11.2 (Continued)

| Basic themes | Organising themes | Global themes |
|---|---|---|
| At first, the therapist was against using Zoom, thinking 'How will it work?' as the most important thing to her is body contact, leading her to think 'We will lose everything' but now having done teletherapy, the therapist realises that remaining at home can feel like a safe place for children and parents, and sessions can even be more focused (DS) | | |
| Screen-to-screen is a platform that the therapist would never have considered using if she not been forced into it because of the global pandemic. However, it has actually enriched her practice and added to her skillset (R) | | |
| Therapist saw new possibilities and became more inventive and creative (T) | | |
| **Concerns and considerations** | | |
| There is a lack of immediate bodily feedback from the children, e.g., holding hands (K) | Lack of bodily cues | The importance of physical interaction |
| Certain techniques may be less suitable in teletherapy, such as Authentic Movement, as there is less kinaesthetic empathy compared to real life (K) | Essentiality of physical contact | |
| Prefers being together in the room for its richness in terms of being able to pick up bodily cues, as it is mentally exhausting trying to pick up cues that are not visible on screen (R) | Difficulty in building the therapeutic relationship | |
| In real life we would have movement - interactional shaping, rhythm, and flow - as sources of information (T) | | |
| Caution against keeping therapy online as physical contact is essential to human life and screen-to-screen can be deeply alienating and lonely (T) | | |
| During this pandemic when bodies are seen as contaminating, it is our responsibility as dance movement therapists to 'put ourselves in the danger zone' since therapists should not run away from problems, but be with them as best we can, in the circumstances (T) | | |
| Depth of work is lost without the passing and sharing of props physically, particularly with ASD (R) | | |
| Teletherapy can be an introduction to the internal world of children with ASD, albeit a chaotic one, but can be hopeless in terms of the therapeutic relationship, if the child is avoidant or hyperactive (T) | | |

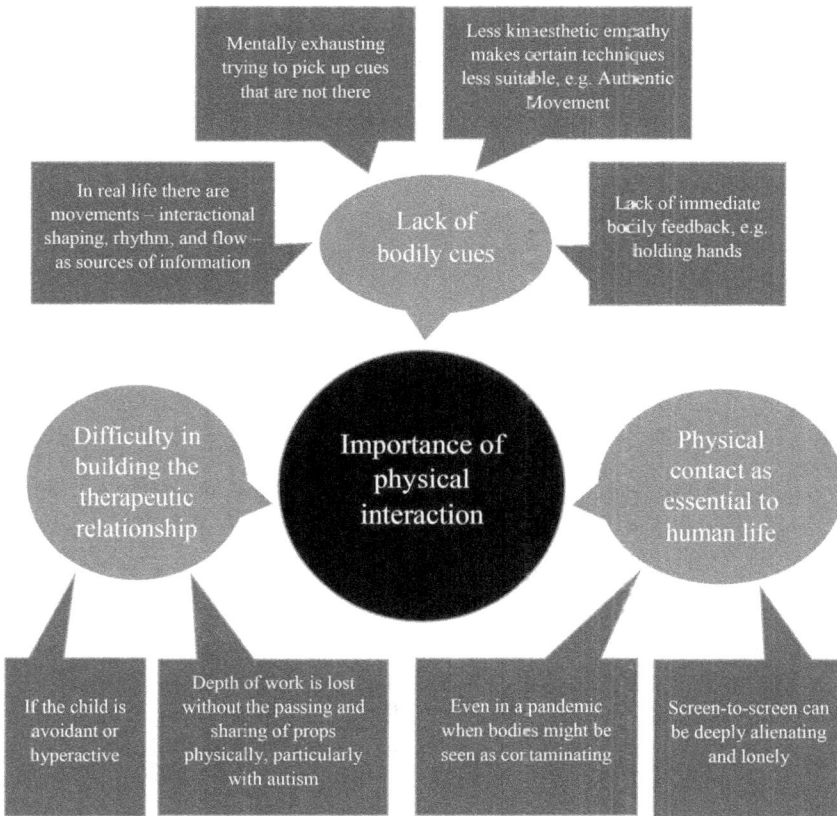

Mentally exhausting trying to pick up cues that are not there

Less kinaesthetic empathy makes certain techniques less suitable, e.g. Authentic Movement

In real life there are movements – interactional shaping, rhythm, and flow – as sources of information

Lack of bodily cues

Lack of immediate bodily feedback, e.g. holding hands

Difficulty in building the therapeutic relationship

Importance of physical interaction

Physical contact as essential to human life

If the child is avoidant or hyperactive

Depth of work is lost without the passing and sharing of props physically, particularly with autism

Even in a pandemic when bodies might be seen as contaminating

Screen-to-screen can be deeply alienating and lonely

*Figure 11.1* The web-like network surrounding a global theme: Importance of physical interaction

To aid in the analysis of the text, as exemplified below in Figure 11.1, for each global theme, a web-like network was drawn. It illustrates how basic themes such as 'Less kinaesthetic empathy, making certain techniques less suitable', and 'Mental exhaustion trying to pick up cues that are not there', can be clustered into an organising theme called 'Lack of bodily cues', which can then be interpreted to relate to the global theme of 'Importance of physical interaction'.

## Discussion

The data were characterised by shared underlying themes and different viewpoints. First, it was helpful to note the two types of teletherapy used: screen-to-screen and telephone. As mentioned by the interview respondents (R, T), texting therapy is another option that exists.

In terms of therapeutic elements or methods in the respondents' work, three global themes were identified: 'Tele-DMP as DMP as usual', 'Tele-DMP as a window', and 'Tele-DMP as a filter'. Therapeutic elements or methods which are helpful in face-to-face DMP with individuals with ASD were used in tele-DMP, including mirroring and attunement, playing, using structure, meeting the clients where they are, music, and 'holding' (Winnicott, 1971), a psychodynamic term referring to how a parent allows their child to express emotion whilst keeping them safe, and how therapists can create this environment for their clients too. Where tele-DMP differed from face-to-face DMP were in the adjustments made, some of which were geared towards maximising the sense of reality through sound, sight, and movement, whether on the part of the client or therapist. There was the use of technological devices to facilitate audio-visual perception that most resembled real life in terms of clarity and synchrony (K), and the use of space in a two-dimensional framework to convey three-dimensional space in reality (DS, K, T). In a shortage of bodily cues, there was the use of aids such as visual art and drawing to visualise thoughts and feelings externally (R, T) and the use of verbal and vocal means to communicate (T). The therapist also mentioned having freedom to move in telephone therapy (T), as in therapy in person. In this sense, these therapeutic methods seemed to serve as a window to reality.

At the same time, the question of 'What is real?' comes to mind in interpreting another cluster of therapeutic methods where tele-DMP seemed to act as a filter to sieve out the distractions in reality. This is exemplified in telephone therapy, which allowed clients to self-reflect without the distractions or pressures of visual stimuli and as such, was 'more defined whilst more remote' (T). In the same vein, focusing on smaller movements such as facial expressions (K) as well as having an anchor for movement, e.g., mindfulness (K), internal reflection (T), verbal checking and understanding (T), and sitting grounded (R), perhaps allowed internal work by 'reducing the frame', a common practice in psychotherapy, as pointed out by a therapist (T). Given these interpretations, in choosing an approach, it is important to consider the needs of the individual with ASD and what is real to them. Similar to how some individuals with ASD may be more comfortable in their home environment for learning (Ameis et al., 2020), likewise they may value the opportunity to minimise difficulties that can occur in face-to-face therapy, e.g. sensory sensitivities and transitioning from place to place. Such stressors may be contributing factors to why a high percentage of carers of individuals with ASD preferred not to return to their daily routines pre-COVID-19, as indicated in a survey in the UK (Pavlopoulou et al., 2020). In this sense, tele-DMP can offer a therapeutic journey that is more sustainable for certain individuals with ASD as a result of less stress for them and their family.

In terms of the outcomes, the global themes of 'Positive feelings', 'Maintenance', and 'New possibilities and development' were identified. Akin to the outcomes in face-to-face DMP, some positive feelings mentioned (DS, K, R) included being happy, playful, excited, and feeling secure, seen, and having a sense of connection (DS, R) which led to increased attendance and new attendees in group therapy (R). Nonetheless, varying attendance rates should be noted as there were different reactions to the screen, including feelings of security but also screen fatigue. These findings were echoed in a study on family-centred tele-DMP with children with autism as there were benefits socially but also challenges as screen interactions were unfamiliar or unmotivating to some (Moo & Ho, 2013). Insofar as tele-DMP was not ideal, it at least served the purpose of maintenance (T) in that clients who continued with tele-DMP were in a better place and were less withdrawn than those who stopped therapy completely. These two global themes seem to highlight the importance of connection during the pandemic, when many may have experienced feeling isolated. Although it remains to be seen if clients will continue to value staying connected in teletherapy post-pandemic, this may be a valuable objective and outcome in therapeutic work. This seems to corroborate the recommendation that children with ASD who were previously engaged with psychotherapy should continue therapy online during the pandemic (Narzisi, 2020).

Additionally, modified ways of working through tele-DMP were found to be helpful for individuals with ASD in novel ways, allowing internal self-reflection (T), creativity, and new possibilities for clients (DS,T), and parents to develop new perspectives (DS). These therapeutic outcomes as a result of the innovation in tele-DMP could speak to its usefulness post-pandemic. They have also resulted in the therapists' seeing new possibilities in tele-DMP and led to therapist development. The sense of therapist and client co-journeying highlights perhaps a connection in the reality of the present moment that is the pandemic.

In terms of concerns and considerations in using tele-DMP with children and adolescents with ASD, the global themes of 'Importance of physical contact', 'The therapeutic space', and 'Future work' were identified. Lack of bodily cues in tele-DMP (K, R, T), difficulty in building the therapeutic relationship (R, T), and the idea of physical contact as essential to human life (T) point to the importance of physical interaction. This need may be most profound during a time of social distancing. Therefore, it is important to consider how DMP can be held in person safely whilst maintaining social distancing. As mentioned by a therapist (T), dance movement therapists have a responsibility to be with problems 'the best we can, in the circumstances', even during a pandemic when 'bodies are seen as contaminating'. Though tele-DMP may be most convenient during periods of pandemic and social distancing, one therapist (T) cautioned against keeping therapy online and viewed physical contact as essential to human life. Hence, although there are a range of telehealth services that may be beneficial for individuals with ASD (Sutherland et al., 2018), interventions calling for physical contact or presence should ideally be conducted in person. The physical presence of the therapist can provide a 'holding' environment therapeutically (Winnicott, 1971) whilst the presence of familiar peers can help motivate children with ASD (Moo & Ho, 2023).

The limitations of using the screen (DS, K, R) and difficulty involving parents (DS) point to the limitations of the screen and possibly home, as a therapeutic 'holding' space. Home may be less conducive for therapy as it is often associated with rest and often, there are scheduling issues, disruptions, and distractions (Moo & Ho, 2023). Moreover, during this period of sudden home confinement, clients and their families may be contending with their relationships with the screen and with each other. This may affect their ability and willingness to engage in screen-to-screen tele-DMP.

Lastly, given the recency of the pandemic at the time of this study, the context of tele-DMP may have been firefighting. More time and planning would have possibly allowed the therapists to bring their work to clients more creatively and push the boundaries of movement (R). It is worth considering the role of movement in tele-DMP, as face to face DMP usually facilitates physical being with and movement together. In tele-DMP, in the absence of physical proximity, the role of movement may be attenuated, or conversely, heightened.

In summary, in choosing an approach in tele-DMP, it is important to consider the needs of the individual with ASD and what is real to them. Simply staying connected with others was a valued therapeutic outcome during the pandemic, and may be a worthwhile objective when using tele-DMP in general. However, there are concerns regarding the sustained and exclusive use of tele-DMP due to its lack of physical interaction. Whilst the limitations of tele-DMP currently are apparent, it may be worth investigating the role of movement in the absence of physical proximity.

## Limitations

Although this study meets the recommended minimum number of participants to infer patterns through thematic analysis (Braun and Clarke, 2013), a larger sample size may have helped generate more data. However, the recency of the pandemic had perhaps meant that a limited number of dance movement therapists had tried using tele-DMP; other dance movement therapists may have not used it for other reasons, which also formed the rationale of this investigation. Although only four dance movement therapists responded to the call to participate in this research, the authors still drew on thematic analysis to identify any meaningful patterns, whilst looking closely at individual texts.

## Conclusion

This study aimed to investigate the use of tele-DMP for children and adolescents with ASD during the COVID-19 pandemic. It demonstrated that tele-DMP presents innovations but also limitations that may be particularly pronounced due to the nature of DMP. Although further planning using this approach may yield different results, at present tele-DMP seems best suited as an interim or adjunct measure due to the distinct advantages of meeting in person.

## Acknowledgements

The authors would like to express their gratitude to the interview respondents: Crista Kwok (Hong Kong), Gemma Ross (the United Kingdom), Jonas Torrance (the United Kingdom), and Sarah dos Santos (based in New Zealand) for sharing their time, expertise, and experience.

## References

Ameis, S.H., Lai, M.C., Mulsant, B.H. and Szatmari, P. (2020) 'Coping, fostering resilience, and driving care innovation for autistic people and their families during the COVID-19 pandemic and beyond', *Molecular Autism*, 11(1), pp. 1–9. 10.1186/s13229-020-00365-y

American Psychiatric Association. (2013) *Diagnostic and statistical manual of mental disorders (5th ed.)*. American Psychiatric Publishing.

Association of Dance Movement Psychotherapy UK (2013). *What is Dance Movement Psychotherapy?* https://admp.org.uk/dance-movement-psychotherapy/what-is-dance-movement-psychotherapy/

Attride-Stirling, J. (2001) 'Thematic networks: An analytic tool for qualitative research', *Qualitative Research*, 1(3), pp. 385–405. 10.1177/146879410100100307.

Aithal, S., Moula, Z., Karkou, V., Karaminis, T., Powell, J., and Makris, S. (2021a). 'A systematic review of the contribution of dance movement psychotherapy towards the well-being of children with autism spectrum disorders', *Frontiers in Psychology*, 12.10.3389/fpsyg.2021.719673.

Aithal, S., Karkou, V., Makris, S., Karaminis, T., and Powell, J. (2021b). 'A dance movement psychotherapy intervention for the wellbeing of children with an autism spectrum disorder: A pilot intervention study', *Frontiers in Psychology*, 1210.3389/fpsyg.2021.588418.

Braun, V. and Clarke, V. (2006) 'Using thematic analysis in psychology', *Qualitative Research in Psychology*, 3, pp. 77–101. 10.1191/1478088706qp063oa.

Braun, V. and Clarke, V. (2013) *Successful qualitative research: A practical guide for beginners*. Sage.

Baudino, L.M. (2010) 'Autism Spectrum Disorder: A Case of Misdiagnosis', *American Journal of Dance Therapy*, 32(2), pp. 113–129. 10.1007/s10465-010-9095-x.

Devereaux, C. (2017) 'Educator perceptions of dance/movement therapy in the special education classroom', *Body, Movement and Dance in Psychotherapy*, 12(1), pp. 50–65. 10.1080/17432979.2016.123801.1.

Lai, M.C., Kassee, C., Besney, R., Bonato, S., Hull, L., Mandy, W., Szatmari, P. and Ameis, S.H. (2019) 'Prevalence of co-occurring mental health diagnoses in the autism population: A systematic review and meta-analysis', *The Lancet Psychiatry*, 6(10), pp. 819–829. 10.1016/S2215-0366(19)30289-5.

Moo, J.T.N and Ho, R.T.H. (2023) 'Benefits and challenges of tele-dance movement psychotherapy with children with autism and their parents', *Digital Health*, 9. 10.1177/20552076231171233

Narzisi, A. (2020) 'Handle the autism spectrum condition during coronavirus (Covid-19) stay at home period: Ten tips for helping parents and caregivers of young children', *Brain Sciences*, 10(4). 10.3390/brainsci10040207.

Partelli, D. (1995) 'Aesthetic listening: Contributions of dance/movement therapy to the psychic understanding of motor stereotypes and distortions in autism and psychosis in childhood and adolescence', *The Arts in Psychotherapy*, 22(3), pp. 241–247. 10.1016/0197-4556(95)00033-2.

Pavlopoulou, G., Wood, R. and Papadopoulos, C. (2020) *Impact of Covid-19 on the experiences of parents and family carers of autistic children and young people in the UK*. London, UK: UCL Institute of Education.

Samaritter, R. and Payne, H. (2017) 'Through the kinaesthetic lens: Observation of social attunement in autism spectrum disorders', *Behavioral Sciences*, 7(1). 10.33 90/bs7010014.

Scharoun, S.M., Reinders, N.J., Bryden, P.J. and Fletcher, P.C. (2014) 'Dance/ movement therapy as an intervention for children with autism spectrum disorders', *American Journal of Dance Therapy*, 36(2), pp. 209–228. 10.1007/s10465-014-9179-0.

Sun, F. (2020) 'For Hong Kong students with special needs, coronavirus pandemic is harming more than just education – it can make their symptoms worse', *South China Morning Post*. https://www.scmp.com/news/hong-kong/education/article/3075217/students-special-needs-hong-kong-coronavirus-pandemic.

Sutherland, R., Trembath, D. and Roberts, J. (2018) 'Telehealth and autism: A systematic search and review of the literature', *International Journal of Speech Language Pathology*, Early Online: 1–13. 10.1080/17549507.2018.1465123.

Takahashi, H., Matsushima, K. and Kato, T. 'The effectiveness of dance/movement therapy interventions for autism spectrum disorder: A systematic review', *American Journal of Dance Therapy*, 41, pp. 55–74 (2019). 10.1007/s10465-019-09296-5.

Torrance, J. (2003) 'Autism, aggression, and developing a therapeutic contract', *American Journal of Dance Therapy*, 25(2), pp. 97–109. http://dx.doi.org.eproxy.lib.hku.hk/10.1023/B:AJOD.0000004757.28220.68.

UNESCO. (2020) *COVID-19 Impact on education*. https://en.unesco.org/covid19/educationresponse.

Winnicott, D. (1971) *Playing and reality*. London: Routledge.

# Appendix

Table A From basic themes to organising themes to global themes

| Basic themes | Organising themes | Global themes |
| --- | --- | --- |
| **Therapeutic elements or methods** | | |
| Seeing what each person needs in the moment and joining them (DS) | Mirroring and attunement/ | Tele-DMP as DMP as usual |
| Working with parents to help parents meet their children where they are at and accept them (DS) | Meeting them where they are | Tele-DMP as a window |
| If you can, observe their movements and reflect (K) | Playing | Tele-DMP as a filter |
| Use household items as props and toys (DS) | Using structure | |
| Playing with sound – listening to sounds and dancing (K) | Holding | |
| Play with emojis as a means of following the children's leads (K) | Music | |
| Using more structured programmes and instructions (K) | Using devices to facilitate audio-visual perception that is more like real life | |
| Chacian Model of introduction, warm up, process, cool down, goodbye (T) | Utilising space in 2D to convey space in reality | |
| Being mindful and letting clients feel safe first, with a 'less is more' approach (K) | Using aids to visualise externally | |
| Recognising integral knowledge in holding the group and holding the individual, even on the screen-to-screen platform (R) | Using verbal and vocal means | |
| Creating safe holding space (R) | Moving freely, more like real life | |
| Managing anxiety (R) | Using devices to reduce the frame | |
| Being with as best we can and not running away from problems or difficult feelings (T) | Working with smaller movements | |
| Use household items as musical instruments (DS) | Having an internal anchor for movement | |
| Rhythmic movement (K) | | |
| Play musical instruments (K) | | |
| Play music from devices (K) | | |
| Hiding self-view in screen-to-screen therapy, to be more like real life, although self-view can be helpful for self-reflexivity (T) | | |
| Utilising space in camera to explore polarities (DS,K) | | |
| Journeying through the space to remind clients that therapist is real as reality becomes less distinct in 2D, so let clients see the space and have a sense of moving and crossing | | |

(Continued)

*Table A* (Continued)

| Basic themes | Organising themes | Global themes |
|---|---|---|
| distance (T) | | |
| Arts and drawing with pen and paper (R) | | |
| Mandala work (T) | | |
| Figures and toys representing feelings and relationships (T) | | |
| Call and response, modulating the voice, dancing with the voice (T) | | |
| Telephone therapy gives the therapist freedom to move (T) | | |
| Using telephone therapy, like text, which is more defined but more remote (T) | | |
| Clients hiding self-view in telephone therapy reduces the frame, encourages internal self-reflection, and is more like real life (T) | | |
| Voice is intimate and encourages internal self-reflection, in telephone therapy (T) | | |
| Responding to clients' small and distinctive movements and gestures (DS) | | |
| Managing parents' expectations by reminding them that little movements are important too (DS) | | |
| Interesting micromovements in facial expressions, e.g., 'happy face' – with clients being more focused and willing to engage as they like electronic things like the camera and feel safer (K) | | |
| Not necessarily big movements (K) | | |
| Mindfulness movement (K) | | |
| Very much sitting in a chair and containing (R) | | |
| At most, breathing, body scan, and grounding in a chair, if clients are in the right environment (R) | | |
| More internal, meditative, and explorative work (T) | | |
| Would only explore how we move through space in 2D with clients who have already done movement together with therapist before in real life (T) | | |

In teletherapy, the scene is set verbally, movements are more in terms of body language (T)
Verbal checking and understanding (T)

## Outcomes

The children were excited and happy to take part (DS)

Adolescents verbalised that they were happy after taking part in sound and movement and imagery exercises (K)

Children were happy to jump around during a time when they had been stuck at home because of the pandemic (K)

Children felt happy and playful following activities utilising space in the camera to explore polarities (K)

New attendees benefited from the layer of security offered by the screen, which created a holding space (R)

The children felt seen in the give and take and sharing of movements (DS)

Each member was acknowledged, and a sense of connection, support, and wellness was fostered through repetitive common movements (DS)

The group helped hold anxiety and created a structure for connecting, sharing, and being with a group (R)

Maintenance: Clients who did teletherapy were in a better place and were less withdrawn than those who stopped therapy altogether (T)

Some were more reserved and preferred to have their cameras turned off (K)

Clients with screen fatigue dropped in number but those who attended did so religiously (R)

Clients' explored internal self-reflection, especially with telephone therapy which is more defined whilst more remote (T)

Using household items as props opened creativity (DS)

It enabled clients to see new possibilities (T)

Parents learned to appreciate little movements (DS)

Children observed the therapist more than other children (K)

At first, the therapist was against using Zoom, thinking 'How will it work?' as the most important thing to her is body contact, ('We will lose everything') but now having done

Positive feelings
Connecting with others
Maintenance of well-being
Different reactions to the screen, resulting in varying attendance rates
Internal self-reflection
Creativity and new possibilities for clients
New perspectives for parents
Dynamics Therapist development

Positive feelings
Maintenance of well-being
New possibilities and development

*(Continued)*

*Table A* (Continued)

| Basic themes | Organising themes | Global themes |
|---|---|---|
| teletherapy, the therapist realises that remaining at home can feel like a safe place for children and parents, and sessions can even be more focused (DS) | | |
| Screen-to-screen is a platform that the therapist would never have considered if she had not been forced into it because of the global pandemic. However, it has actually enriched her practice and added to her skillset (R) | | |
| The therapist saw new possibilities and became more inventive and creative (T) | | |
| **Concerns and considerations** | | |
| There is a lack of immediate bodily feedback from the children, e.g., holding hands (K) | Lack of bodily cues | Importance of physical contact |
| Certain techniques may be less suitable in teletherapy, such as Authentic Movement, as there is less kinaesthetic empathy compared to real life (K) | Essentiality of physical contact | The therapeutic space |
| In real life we would have movement - interactional shaping, rhythm, and flow - as sources of information (T) | Difficulty in building the therapeutic relationship | Future work |
| Prefers being together in the room for its richness in terms of being able to pick up bodily cues, as it is mentally exhausting trying to pick up cues that are not visible on screen (R) | Limitations of using the screen | |
| Caution against keeping therapy online as physical contact is essential to human life and screen-to-screen can be deeply alienating and lonely (T) | Time to plan creatively | |
| During this pandemic when bodies are seen as contaminating, it is our responsibility as DMPs to 'put ourselves in the danger zone' since therapists should not run away from problems, but be with them as best we can, in the circumstances (T) | Difficulty involving parents | |
| Depth of work is lost without the passing and sharing of props physically, particularly with ASD (R) | | |
| Teletherapy can be an introduction to the internal world of children with ASD, albeit a chaotic one, but can be hopeless in terms of the therapeutic relationship, if the child is avoidant or hyperactive (T) | | |
| Some children come too close to the camera (K) | | |
| Clients who were previously moving in therapy in person were in contrast, uncomfortable moving when in their chairs or bed. The therapist was uncomfortable too for those | | |

reasons (R)
Need time to think about how to bring the work creatively if we go into lockdown again (R)
Parents may be unready to sacrifice their time and may not be comfortable with the screen (DS)
Parents may not be prepared to take a step back to listen to their children and see them with different eyes as it is a big step to see every little thing as significant (DS)

Chapter 12

# From Music Therapist to Action Research Designer

## A Narrative Account

*Grazia Ragone, Emeline Brulé, Kate Howland, and Judith Good*

## Introduction

Participation has become a key element in the development of technology to ensure its fair use (McCarthy and Wright, 2015). This is particularly true for assistive technology, which has a notoriously low uptake rate due to a combination of factors, including its often-cumbersome design, high price, and/or it not meeting users' needs or desires. In response to this, human-computer interaction (HCI) scholars have proposed a range of participatory methods for design and have even trained users in design methodologies in a Do-It-Yourself or Do-It-Together approach, leading to a growth in networks, organisations, and tools to support the development of technologies by disabled people, or disability professionals such as therapists (Hook et al., 2014). It is however difficult to bridge these two bodies of expertise, and even more difficult to ensure that the novel tools and interventions are appropriately tested (Brule et al., 2016). In this chapter, we outline one way to approach this issue: the interdisciplinary training of a music therapist, who, during her practice in music therapy, designed a touchless system that supports the music-making activity of autistic children with the whole body, and has subsequently undertaken academic research on the design and evaluation of this tool (Ragone et al., 2020).

Music therapy leverages music to achieve developmental, adaptive, and rehabilitative goals in the areas of psychosocial, cognitive, and sensory motor skills (Hurt-Thaut, 2009). It is becoming more common in educational services for autistic children, and those with behavioural and learning disabilities. Music is a distinctive area to assess perception, emotion, and other physiological reactions and neural circuitry of autistic people (Quintin, 2019), which is moreover enjoyable. However, for children who experience multiple disabilities, using a traditional musical instrument can be difficult, and can therefore prevent them from benefiting from the intervention; this is the first area in which technological innovation could be useful. Moreover, there are significant debates around understanding and measuring the impact

DOI: 10.4324/9781003201656-16

of music therapy on children; this is the second area in which technologies could be useful. These two goals cannot be achieved without the participation of music therapists themselves, but existing research rarely includes them as active participants (Ragone et al., 2021). This chapter provides an example and some explanations as to why participation is difficult, and outlines design opportunities for music therapists and technology researchers to pursue.

## Study Approach

Analysing the researcher's experience is a way to understand the conditions of the production of knowledge, and to generate a qualitative and interpretative understanding of the activities they aim to change. This critical reflection on the researcher's experience (Mortari, 2015), which is crucial in action research, can employ several methodological approaches, such as narrative research, heuristic inquiry, or auto-ethnography (Andrews et al., 2013; Roth, 2005).

According to Schön (1983), the sum of what a practitioner knows is more significant than what they can articulate, a tacit knowledge that can be useful in research collaborations but is difficult to codify. The experience of our first author, as a music therapist first and a researcher later, represents here the research material as qualitative accounts written by the researcher, of her background and experiences past and present in the form of narrative research. This account is contextualised within her notes, in the shape of vignettes and the relevant literature, to highlight relevant methodological and theoretical insights into how her practice changed over time. While this type of narrative research is often conducted by the researcher alone, we have found it useful to collaborate on this account as a form of collective meaning–making that can further reveal the challenges of practitioner-led action research from the perspective of more senior academics.

### Background: Music Therapy at the Crossroads of Music and Health

*I have loved music since I can remember. When I was an adolescent, studying music was always the dominant option during conversations with my parents. For my bachelor's degree in Systematic Musicology, which I obtained in 2004, I delineated a path in my degree dissertation towards music therapy, which was still unknown and considered unusual in this context. Although different music therapy programs were operating in Italy, where I was living, there was a substantial difference between music-making approaches for practitioners in musicology and music therapy. Music therapy uses music to address non-musical goals, which can explain why it is absent from the musicologists' academic curricula, which is focused instead on the theoretical aspects of music. I completed an internship at the Maggiore Hospital in Parma (Italy), working with patients with Alzheimer's Disease. Then, I moved to Rome to complete my master's degree in Music and Art therapy. Finally, I continued my practice at the San Filippo Neri Hospital with a group of people with Alzheimer's and Parkinson's Diseases. I could write at length about the extreme emotions of working with persons finding harbour in singing yesteryear lyrics from their youth as they were losing the ability to form short-term memories—as previously described by* Sacks (2008) *for instance.*

Music is a relational experience, but this was not necessarily emphasised in Grazia's musicology studies. Music therapy was firmly kept beyond its boundaries, as a care practice. Care practices are often undervalued, perceived as messy and requiring little skill (Mol et al., 2010). Music therapy is similarly at the periphery of medicine. Music therapists focus on experiences that medical professionals may not have the time to address: the difficult emotions, being there rather than treating and healing. It is with this background that:

*I was then employed by the Rome city council, working in primary schools with autistic children in 2006. My approach to music therapy with autistic children was guided by my mentors: first a psychoanalytical orientation (*Benenzon, 1981*) with a later turn to a humanistic and psychodynamic one (*Stefani and Guerra-Lisi, 2006*). I ran weekly individual and group sessions and, by rotation, sessions with mixed groups of autistic and allistic[1] children to support social integration.*

According to *DSM-5* (APA, 2013), Autism Spectrum Disorders(ASD) are characterised by two core features: deficits in social communication and social interaction, and restricted, repetitive patterns of behaviour, interests, or activities. Additionally, and relevant to music therapy practice, Bhat and colleagues (2020) report that a significant percentage (87%) of the autistic population have motor difficulties, ranging from an atypical gait (gross motor skills) to difficulties with handwriting (fine motor skills). Other studies (Wilson et al., 2018) have demonstrated that autistic children present motor differences such as clumsiness, abnormal motor coordination, postural insecurity, and weak performance in standardised testing of motor functioning. Despite their robust presence and their negative impact on learning and social interaction (Green et al., 2009), motor issues are not considered a core trait of autism. Music therapy is attractive to autism practitioners because they often seek to support autistic children in developing social communication and interaction skills, and in some cases, motor functioning. Music therapy helps in supporting joint attention, social reciprocity, and nonverbal and verbal communication (Srinivasan and Bhat, 2013).

### Developing as a Music Therapist with Autistic Children

After five years of working for the Rome city council as a music therapist and as a trainer for teachers to deliver music therapy sessions in various mainstream schools, the primary aim of Grazia's work was to integrate autistic children in their classrooms. Below are excerpts from her notes at the time, reflecting how Grazia and her colleagues conceptualised and assessed the impact of music therapy. To protect the confidentiality of the children mentioned in this paper, all the names used are pseudonyms.

> As the small group of 6 floats into the room, where all the musical instruments are placed onto the floor, I welcome them with a melodic song calling each one's name. This is the 3rd session with the same group. The chosen instruments of the day are primarily rhythmic and two melodics. When Manuel arrives, he sits apart, not on the spot I assigned for him and far from the rest of the group sitting in the shape of a circle. I leave him watching us, although I continue to keep him in through gaze. We all play a 4/4 rhythm while I keep singing. Finally, he stood up and sat closer to the group, still not on his spot and apart from the group.

At the time, the only way Grazia and her colleagues could evaluate the trend of the session and the therapeutic goals was via a thorough written report composed of summative feedback recorded during and after the session. Most of the notes came from the individual diary that therapists kept and could consequently share regularly with the rest of the team, made up of parents, teachers, psychologists, and other relevant professionals. In the analysis, Grazia always looked at specific features of joint behaviour, communication and interaction that would be relevant to the aims of the therapeutic process while also being comparable across different sessions. She noted simple, relatively unambiguous behaviour that can be coded, such as movements and face behaviour and rhythmic activity. In this third session, Manuel, for the first time, clearly showed his willingness to be engaged in our way of making music as a group. The overall intervention lasted 18 months including school holidays. Below is another extract of Grazia's notes from four months later:

> Today we had a group of 8 children working with Manuel. In the room, I placed only two rhythmic instruments. On their arrival, after the welcome song, I asked them to move freely following me while I was playing a simple 4/4 rhythm. They were all synced after we started playing the 'Identity beat' game where one child per time had to move naturally, and the rest of the group followed them copying the movements. Children were having lots of fun, and when it came to his turn, Manuel was pleased that everyone else was following him; he was smiling, laughing, and

*jumping, experimenting with new, unusual movements, checking that everyone else was following him. Manuel still averted his gaze.*

*After a couple of individual sessions of music therapy, he started better articulating his words and started to sing and show his talent to sing in tune with any melody he heard. His echolalic expression became a strength.*

The therapeutic goal was initially to support Manuel to develop his vocal sounds into spoken words through music therapy. But, by the end of the academic year, he showed great musical ability and the rest of his classroom learnt how to relate to him and respect the moments when he was upset or struggling with social demands. His verbal communication dramatically improved, and he was able to articulate specific requests. After a few sessions, he began to make sparse eye contact and interact, first with Grazia as his therapist and then with other children in his class. He loved to express himself through singing with the rest of the group but never showed any interest in playing musical instruments; sometimes he was even bothered by percussive instruments. Grazia often felt that he considered musical instruments to be intrusive. Even with the piano, every time he was asked to play, he would never press the keys for long.

### Towards the Transition

*While I was practising as a therapist, I was constantly researching new ways, through music, to address therapeutic goals with Manuel and other children like him. I had the feeling that music therapy, although having high potential for autistic child users, had a few limitations too. During my years of training and practice, I continuously exchanged opinions with other therapists and musicians and artists every time the opportunity arose to talk about music and its potential. I was still searching for new ways to practise music therapy and tailor it for larger groups, when in 2008, I came across a group of researchers at the Italian National Council of Research (CNR) in Pisa (Italy). At the CNR's developers' team, I put forward my idea of developing a new tool to practise music therapy, a contactless, invisible musical instrument, which at the outset I named ConTatto, that could translate each gesture into a sound, and a sequence of harmonic motions could generate a melody. ConTatto was implemented as a standalone application. It provided an immersive sensorial experience for the children who could feel themselves as being the source of sound in their free movements in space. We specifically designed a room at the CNR where there were no distractions, with white walls and with all cables hidden. The ConTatto system was based on an Apple Macintosh computer and consisted of a video camera, connected through a Firewire digitiser, that allowed a latency of only one frame in the video processing path. The algorithms detected and extrapolated features from the child, such as spatial position, arm and leg angles, and speed, while an operator - in addition to the therapist - could link these features to sounds synthesised in real-time, following an agreed schema defined by the therapist. The technology presented a few limitations though, such as the influence of the ambient light to avoid shadows that could also affect the precision of motion detection. Also, the presence of another technician who needed to control the system, following my guidance as therapist, could represent a distraction for the child. Additionally, when there were last minute changes according to the child's reactions, it was difficult to exchange that information between myself and the technician, avoiding the child's involvement. At the time, I was not even aware of the existence of the HCI world.*

HCI focuses on how people interact with computers and evaluates the extent to how computers are or are not developed for effective interaction with human beings. As a natural implication from its name, HCI entails the connection between the human user, the computer itself, and how they interact together. In the last decades, the use of technologies in the HCI field has expanded the ways people can make and experience music (Ragone et al., 2020). This led to the dramatic increase of motion sensing technologies that have become pervasive in so many fields including music therapy that needed to adapt itself.

*However, at that time, I was still unconcerned that I was crossing the road between being a therapist and becoming a researcher in HCI. It took years to go through the process. While I still was a therapist, I always tried to stay informed by academic research and took any idea that could shape and ameliorate my practice. I was aware of how this kind of partnership could promote the significance, practicability, and value of research and the potential efficacy of care while being a therapist.*

Grazia was interested in research on motor skills before becoming a researcher. Gestures bring both semantic and pragmatic content to communication (Capone and McGregor, 2004). de Marchena et al. (2019) showed how autistic participants have nonverbal tactics for regulating conversational dynamics to enable conversational turn-taking. The same study demonstrated that motoric features were associated with individual autistic symptoms. These theoretical backgrounds and other studies (Torres and Donnellan, 2015) which highlighted the importance of motor differences in the early years as moderators to predict a future diagnosis of autism led her to focus her attention on the motor aspect in the design of the new musical tool. Musical gestures and body motion in music have recently been the focus of extensive interdisciplinary research from different disciplines such as musicology, cognitive psychology, neurology, and computer science (Godøy and Leman, 2010). New approaches to embodied music cognition (Leman, 2008) offered new perspectives and required a rethink of the relationship between the human body and musical experience.

*During my master's degree in the School of Psychology at the University of Sussex, I analysed the first dataset collected, using an updated version of ConTatto, in a pilot study conducted in Italy with a group of 10 autistic children, aged 6 to 10 years old. It was a decisive step in the transition from being a practitioner to becoming a researcher. As a music therapist, I could not produce intelligible data reflecting the efficacy of my work. I thought technology could provide this data, which would in turn allow for clearer communication between researchers and practitioners. But I quickly realised that wearing both hats ran the risk that one role would become dominant. As a practitioner, I see my main goal as contributing to the client's well-being. In contrast, as a researcher, I see my goal as describing, predicting, evaluating, and understanding. Before identifying myself as a researcher, I had to bring the two perspectives together.*

### The Change in Perspective

*I recall, during my practice, my experience with nonspeaking children whose body language was often more eloquent than words. As a music therapist, I was struggling to find an objective way to collect data and document my studies to make a wider contribution to knowledge. I needed to explore new methodologies and approaches to children and data collection when new visions were opening promising avenues towards new technologies. At the time myself and the team I was working with were still unaware of the existence of the Kinect for Xbox 360, which was subsequently presented in June 2009, it looked like the future of technology and the answer to my need in documenting a mixed-method approach.*

*For my PhD in HCI at Sussex, I wanted to learn more about why music therapy was effective, and the role of movement in this. I also still wanted to develop ConTatto (which evolved into OSMoSIS), the tool I had envisioned when working with Manuel and with other children for whom traditional musical instruments led to frustration over not being able to make a nice piece of music as well as not being able to properly hold some instruments. In addition, I learned of research showing that autistic children might lack full awareness of their bodies which also affects their ability to self-regulate (Schauder et al., 2015). I then focused on ways of promoting self-recognition of own-body movements providing an interactive and playful space to enhance perception, action, and self-awareness skills.*

We designed an HCI system, OSMoSIS (Observation of Social Motor Synchrony in an Interactive System), which allows the sonification of dyadic coordinated human rhythmic activity and uses the Microsoft Kinect to accurately track and process body movements to enhance the child's body awareness unobtrusively. The name chosen, OSMoSIS, reflected the aim of a user-centric approach, where a process of gradual assimilation of ways to interact with others and express and communicate through sounds and body movements happens. OSMoSIS aims to enhance children's perception and provide bodily consistency through a simultaneous cross-modal mapping of body motion qualities from bodily movement to sounds. OSMoSIS, using Microsoft's Kinect camera, is not intrusive for the child and generates an interacting environment in response to the child's movements. One of the advantages, a requirement for its development, was to record the movements pattern of children to reflect their engagement during the session. This signed a significant advancement due to the adopted Kinect technology's ability to analyse in detail the 25 body joints of the child while they interact in the interactive space. Also, it addressed one of the needs of the therapists to generate intelligible data reflecting the efficacy of the interventions.

OSMoSIS was designed to prioritise ease-of-use and simplicity, addressing one of the significant issues encountered in the music therapy practice where some instruments, such as the guitar, can sometimes be too complicated for those with cognitive or physical impairments, limiting their scope for expression (Magee, 2006). OSMoSIS represents a new way to practice music therapy where children do not encounter barriers to music-making but express themselves through sounds as a vehicle of interaction, social and emotional development without the necessary involvement of verbal communication, aim of the music therapy.

With OSMoSIS, Grazia has run three studies with three groups of ten children each. Each study had a similar design in terms of interaction where, in four 1:1 sessions, the researcher proposed four movements associated with four sounds with specific characteristics. In each session, Grazia presented four movements (hopping, marching, waving arms, moving the whole body) associated to four sounds (waterdrop, drum, guitar, marimba) to the children who were asked to mimic her movements. The sessions were divided into two conditions, where Grazia proposed the same movements with no auditory feedback in the first condition or associated with sounds in the second condition. For instance, the 'hopping' movement was associated with the waterdrop or the 'marching' with the drum. In summary, we noticed a higher level of interaction between the children and the facilitator with the system active. The main difference between traditional music therapy and the new music interdisciplinary HCI approach consisted in the absence of mediators such as instruments to free up children's expression and creativity. With OSMoSIS, children's bodies act as musical instruments and the more they move, the more sounds happen around them. The lack of the embodied phenomenon that traditional instruments offer needs to be weighed against the potential for the user to participate actively in making sound within a therapeutic communication. With this new perspective, gestures are not seen as a means to control musical instruments which generate sounds but rather as a further significant agent to the formation of musical meaning.

*Today, with Kinect, my research is still ongoing, and it is not the goal of this paper to offer comprehensive evidence about the efficacy of the approach with OSMoSIS. However, my studies and analysis so far have identified promising benefits, and several avenues for further research.*

### Advantages and Disadvantages

The first author's transition from practice to academia required her to move away from applying existing theories, waive some aesthetic principles regarding the choice of sound, and to following scientific methods, starting from measurable predictions, testing them through empirical studies, and finally to objectively determining whether the results support the hypotheses. One of the limitations associated with integrating technology into the new music therapy approach is often a lesser aesthetic musical experience than with acoustic instruments, since sound is generated by MIDI sounds triggered by a switch or a sensor. Traditional musical instruments elicit evocative capabilities due to their multisensory capacities, encompassing several senses such as sight, touch, and smell in addition to sound. This represents a significant limitation for music therapists for whom the search for aesthetic and harmonic properties in sounds is always an important challenge in music making. Also, even more when designing for autistic users, the choice of sound features such as pitch, timbre, and dynamic should be very accurate because of heightened auditory processing in autistic people (Heaton, 2003). In the OSMoSIS design process, it took a long time to find specific sound features to match with simple gestures and which were pleasurable and not difficult to process for autistic users. After the first study we refined sounds as we noticed some sounds were not well-suited to our users.

*Before running the study, I asked to know everything about each child and their experience with particular sounds, but no warning was given to me about any specific issue. I began the data collection with Flo using the guitar sound, and he started interacting with me straight away, mimicking my movements and displaying enjoyment in what he was doing through smiles, eye contact and verbal utterances. The second sound was the 'water flow' associated with a sweeping motion, with the arms pretending to pull at the water. I was showing my arms moving backward and inward when suddenly Flo withdraw himself, moving toward the corner. His face expression became sad with lowered eyelids, downcast eyes and slanting inner eyebrows. I soon interrupted my exercise and switched off the OSMoSIS software which was still generating flowing water sounds according to my movements. Flo asked me to go back to his class. The day after, parents reported to the SENCo that Flo had previously had an upsetting experience while he was experiencing outdoor activities at the river. For the following studies, we used this experience to improve the sound quality and were careful to ask each parent for any suggestions about the use of specific sounds with their children.*

Therefore, the control of sound, the choice of colour, and purposeful design are essential components in designing a setting for autistic children due to their different sensitivities to the environment. In addition, attention to the sound features would be essential to design therapeutical settings, to avoid causing distress or anxiety to participants. Also, the use of technology in clinical practice remains a topic that has been insufficiently researched. A lack of training in the appropriate use of technology in music therapy and access to technology equipment remain the most significant barriers for music therapists. An interchange between researchers and practitioners could establish a framework for developing technologies that can be tailored and used to a client's benefit within clinical care. Each field of practice has its own requirements for matching the user's needs to the technology's features. For instance, music therapists working with adults with neurologic conditions have reported that technology has improved arm movement in people with hemiplegia (Paul and Ramsey, 1998) as well as being useful in facilitating active participation in therapy (Nagler, 1998). Other studies (Hunt et al., 2004) also outline the value of technology in motivating adolescents to engage in therapy. OSMoSIS, with its autism-centric approach, seems to respond to the needs of autistic people; they are able to gain awareness of their bodies through sounds that react in real-time to their movements, supporting their self-regulation.

### Conclusion

Technology design's key success in music therapy needs to be user-centred, addressing client's needs. Although acoustic instruments will still be the preferred tools for music therapists, these instruments cannot always support complex physical needs in such a flexible way.

Although communication between practice and academia still results in largely unresolved issues in design research, technology can provide opportunities promoting the interchange of knowledge and abilities. This narrative research chapter has shown the usefulness of collaboration and cooperation as a form of collective meaning–making that further reveals the challenges of practitioner-led action.

From the stakeholders' perspective, we suggest designing users' tools and testing theories as a collaborative process that aims for transdisciplinary understanding. However, it would also be helpful to bridge the two bodies of expertise of academics and practitioners, allowing appropriate testing of novel tools and interventions. This chapter has outlined one conceivable way to approach the issue: interdisciplinary therapist training.

The advantage of technology, in providing automatic or manual post-processing and mapping data to a model, is that it makes it easier to develop and share evidence-based practice, potentially leading to a good research-practice partnership.

## Note

1   Allistic is based on the Greek word 'allos', meaning 'other', just as 'autos' (in 'autism') means 'self'. The term is widely accepted by the autistic community in opposition to "neurotypical" which implies that someone is intrinsically better or worse. Also, in this work, we use identity-first language (e.g., autistic people) as opposed to person-first language (e.g., people with autism) based on established or emerging preferences within the autistic communities.

## References

Andrews, M., Squire, C. and Tamboukou, M. (2013) *Doing narrative research* (2nd edition). London: SAGE Publications Ltd.

American Psychiatric Association (2013) *Diagnostic and statistical manual of mental disorders* (5th ed., Text Revision).

Benenzon, R.O. (1981) *Music therapy manual*. C.C. Thomas, pp. 1–158.

Bhat, A.N. (2020) 'Is motor impairment in autism spectrum disorder distinct from developmental coordination disorder? A report from the SPARK Study', *Physical Therapy*, 100(4), pp. 633–644.

Brule, E., Bailly, G., Brock, A., Valentin, F., Denis, G. and Jouffrais, C. (2016) 'MapSense: MultiSensory interactive maps for children living with visual impairments', Proceedings of the 2016 CHI Conference on Human Factors in Computing Systems, pp. 445–457.

Capone, N.C. and McGregor, K.K. (2004) 'Gesture development: A review for clinical and research practices', *Journal of Speech, Language, and Hearing Research*, 47, pp. 173–186.

de Marchena, A., Kim, E.S., Bagdasarov, A., Parish-Morris, J., Maddox, B.B., Brodkin, E.S. and Schultz, R.T. (2019) 'Atypicalities of gesture form and function in autistic adults', *Journal of Autism and Developmental Disorders*, 49(4), pp. 1438–1454.

Godøy R.I. and Leman, M.(2010) *Musical gestures: Sound, movement and meaning*. Routledge.

Green, D., Charman, T., Pickles, A., Chandler, S., Loucas, T., Simonoff, E., et al. (2009) 'Impairment in movement skills of children with autistic spectrum disorders', *Developmental Medicine and Child Neurology*, 51(4), pp. 311–316.

Heaton, P. (2003) 'Pitch memory, labelling and disembedding in autism', *J Child Psychol Psychiatry*, 2003(44), pp. 543–551.

Hook, J., Verbaan, S., Durrant, A., Olivier, P. and Wright, P. (2014) 'A study of the challenges related to DIY assistive technology in the context of children with disabilities', Proceedings of the 2014 Conference on Designing Interactive Systems, pp. 597–606.

Hunt, L., Eagle, L. and Kitchen, P. (2004) 'Balancing marketing education and information technology: Matching needs or needing a better match?' *Journal of Marketing Education – Journal of Market Education*, 26, pp. 75–88.

Hurt-Thaut, C. (2009) 'Clinical practice in music therapy', in S. Hallam, I. Cross and M. Thaut (eds.) *The Oxford handbook of music psychology*. Oxford University Press, pp. 503–514.

Leman, M. (2008) *Embodied music cognition and mediation technology*. MIT Press.

Magee, W.L. (2006) 'Electronic technologies in clinical music therapy: A survey of practice and attitudes', *Technology and Disability*, 18(3), pp. 139–146.

McCarthy, J. and Wright, P. (2015) *Taking [a]part: The politics and aesthetics of participation in experience-centered design*. Cambridge, Massachusetts: The MIT Press.

Mol, A., Moser, I. and Pols, J. (2010) 'Care in practice: On tinkering in clinics, homes and farms', *Care in Practice*, 8.

Mortari, L. (2015) 'Reflectivity in research practice: An overview of different perspectives', *International Journal of Qualitative Methods*. 10.1177/160940691561 8045.

Nagler, J. (1998) 'Digital music technology in music therapy practice', in C. Tomaino (ed.) *Clinical applications of music in neurologic rehabilitation*, pp. 41–49.

Paul, S. and Ramsey, D. (1998) 'The effects of electronic music-making as a therapeutic activity for improving upper extremity active range of motion', *Occupational Therapy International*, 5, pp. 223–237.

Quintin, E.-M. (2019) 'Music-evoked reward and emotion: Relative strengths and response to intervention of people with ASD', *Frontiers in Neural Circuits*, 13, p. 49. 10.3389/fncir.2019.00049.

Ragone, G., Good, J. and Howland, K.L. (2020) OSMoSIS | Proceedings of the 2020 ACM Interaction Design and Children Conference: Extended Abstracts. IDC '20: Proceedings of the 2020 ACM Interaction Design and Children Conference. https://doi-org.ezproxy.sussex.ac.uk/10.1145/3397617.3397838.

Ragone, G., Good, J. and Howland, K. (2021) 'How technology applied to music therapy and sound-based activities addresses motor and social skills in autistic children', *Multimodal Technologies and Interaction*, 5(3), p. 11.

Roth, W.-M. (2005) *Auto/biography and auto/ethnography: praxis of research method*. Rotterdam: Sense.

Sacks, O. (2008) *Musicophilia: Tales of music and the brain*. Vintage Books.

Schauder, K.B., Mash, L.E., Bryant, L.K. and Cascio, C.J. (2015) 'Interoceptive ability and body awareness in autism spectrum disorder', *Journal of Experimental Child Psychology*, 131, pp. 193–200.

Schön, D. (1983) *The reflective practitioner: How professionals think in action*. New York: Basic Books.

Stefani, G. and Guerra-Lisi, S. (2006) 'Globalità dei Linguaggi', Manuale di MusicArTerapia, Carocci, Roma.

Srinivasan, S.M. and Bhat, A.N. (2013) 'A review of "music and movement" therapies for children with autism: Embodied interventions for multisystem development', *Frontiers in Integrative Neuroscience*, 2013(7), p. 22.

Torres, E.B. and Donnellan, A.M. (2015) 'Editorial for research topic "Autism: The movement perspective"', *Frontiers in Integrative Neuroscience*, 9, p. 12.

Wilson, R.B., McCracken, J.T., Rinehart, N.J. and Jeste, S.S. (2018) 'What's missing in autism spectrum disorder motor assessments?', *Journal of Neurodevelopmental Disorders*, 10.

# Chapter 13

# Attunement and the Nonverbal Autistic Child

## A Multi-Disciplinary Perspective

*Jeannie Lewis*

## Introduction

Nonverbal and minimally verbal young autistic people have been identified as "the neglected end of the spectrum" (Tager-Flusberg and Kasari, 2013, p1). We know little about the aetiology, experience, therapy, and outcomes of being nonverbal or minimally verbal in autism (Interagency Autism Coordinating Committee, 2011), but we do know it is common with at least 30% affected (Tager-Flusberg et al., 2005). It has been commonly assumed that the severity of a learning disability drives the lack of acquisition or use of speech in autistic children. Estimated rates of learning disability in the autistic population vary widely, they have decreased with increased diagnosis and broadening of diagnostic criteria. Baio et al. (2018) in a large (n = 3,714) US study reported 31% had an IQ below 70, 25% between 71–85, and 44% were in the average or above average range (IQ > 85). However, not all those who do not acquire spoken language have low nonverbal IQ scores (Munson et al., 2008) and some have good receptive language abilities and nonverbal abilities (Rapin et al., 2009). It is increasingly clear there is considerable heterogeneity in cognitive and linguistic skills among nonverbal and minimally verbal autistic children and no single underlying mechanism that explains why some children do not learn to, or choose to, speak (Tager-Flusberg and Kasari, 2013).

This complexity of function and causation in verbalisation in autism is illustrated well by Fletcher-Watson and Happe's (2018) critique of the autism spectrum metaphor which they argue reduces the heterogeneity of autism to a linear continuum from the 'highest functioning' autistic person to the 'lowest' functioning autistic person. Instead, verbal function is better seen within the context of a multidimensional 'constellation' of strengths and difficulties representing complex variability within the autistic population.

The reasons for an autistic person being nonverbal therefore vary recently we have started to hear from nonverbal autistic people themselves. In *The Reason Why I Jump,* the author Naoki Higashida (2013), himself a nonverbal autistic person, attempts to help us understand the sensory world of non-speaking autistic people. The book provides stunning insights into his

DOI: 10.4324/9781003201656-17

nonverbal world and refutes the assumption that verbal ability equals intelligence. This also has parallels with Gardener's (1983) concept of there being multiple intelligences rather than it being a single construct. In *The Reason Why I Jump* Higashida sets out his hope that the book will explain 'what's going on in the minds of people with autism'. The 2020 film *The Reason Why I Jump* (dir Jerry Rothwell) takes viewers into the lives of five nonverbal autistic individuals living across four continents. The book and the film in complementary ways provide a powerful testament to the fact that a lack of speech does not equate with a lack of thought.

Through these works and the identification of nonverbalism as a neglected area in autism research, there is increasing interest in this core experience of many autistic people and how best to provide help and support, if needed. This chapter focusses on the ability and value of dramatherapy and other therapies in enabling, through the process of attunement, nonverbal and minimally verbal autistic children to develop, communicate and process therapeutically their own narratives.

## Study Approach

The chapter's aim is to explore interaction between dramatherapy and nonverbal or minimally verbal autistic children in therapy through the lens of attunement theory. The methodology adopted here is a case study design (Widdowson, 2011). The format is a series of three complementary descriptive and illustrative clinical vignettes of my work as a dramatherapist with nonverbal or minimally verbal autistic children. The themes emerging from these case studies are explored through diverse arts therapies literature and in relation to discussions with non-arts therapists engaged with the same client group. In this way the centrality of the role of attunement in effecting successful therapy, whatever its modality, is explored.

### Case study 1: Adam's story[1] – *The Big and the Little Car and the Little Car Hiding*

*I first observed Adam in class in Year 1 aged six. He had been described as being aggressive by the class team and I saw a pattern of hitting out or knocking things over. I offered play opportunities in the classroom but, while he acknowledged my presence, these were not accepted by him in that setting. It was clear that it would not be helpful to offer further intervention where he was already feeling overloaded. I invited him and his 1:1 assistant to visit the dramatherapy room and set the room up in a way that I hoped would interest him with a variety of different play offers including toys and art materials. I created a social story with photos about the room and asked his 1:1 to share the story with him before the session.*

*When Adam came to the therapy space, he looked around the space and went to play. He selected the cars as play objects and made them crash. He added cars with sirens that came to help. From a distance, I reflected on what was happening by using words and adding sounds using musical instruments. I took pictures of the sessions and the toys he played with and added them to the social storybook. I introduced words into our play that reflected what he was doing: 'more', 'stop', 'finished'. He noticed me do this but did not use the words himself. I initiated a game of 'where's … ?', hiding and revealing. Adam engaged with this and laughed at the surprise reveals. He allowed touch and we drew around his hands and feet. We looked in a mirror at our separate selves and together. At one point, he took the mirror and was interested in using it to look at himself and around the room. I understood this as analogous to a developmental step towards communication, observing the other.*

*Over our sessions, Adam began to create a play sequence with the cars that were repeated. The story was about two cars being squashed by a ball and two cars coming to rescue them. The same cars were used each time. The narrative was played out using simple sounds, engine sounds, a siren or a warning sound. I echoed these sounds using my voice and the musical instruments. He accepted this and looked to me to restart if I stopped. It felt like we were beginning to play together and communicating through this play. I took photos of the different sections of the story and shared them with him using the simple sounds and words that went with them. He recognised the story in photo form and was able to connect the images with the play and the musical sounds. A second narrative developed about a big and a small car, and a little car hiding. There were moments of calm in the sessions, in which we blew bubbles. He said 'up', and I sat him on my shoulders. It felt safe and calm in the sessions. He showed pleasure by laughing and engaging in play. There was a sense of connection between us. Our eye contact increased. Together we had attuned the therapy space and the content of sessions to enable bidirectional communication.*

## Analysis

The key themes emerging from the process cluster into two sequential phases. First, building rapport, establishing the therapeutic space, and preparing the child and therapist for a therapeutic interaction. Second, the importance of a repeated structure/pattern within the session and a secure connection between sessions to build a trusting therapeutic relationship and constructive exchange. Taken together, my analysis at the time was that we were working with a developmental approach building the early steps of communication, and showing that communication was worthwhile. Before training, as a dramatherapist I read *The Silent Child Exploring the World of Children Who Do Not Speak* by Laurent Danon-Boileau (2001) which describes his treatment of six young nonverbal people. On my first read, I questioned the rigidity of his Kleinian interpretations of play; as a therapist, I have found that it is easy to fall into a trap of over-interpretation as well as under-interpretation.

With Adam, I tried to describe and reflect, I used a narrative approach, sometimes in the third person. I tried not to assume a relationship. I was direct and simple. There were times when the symbolic content of the play felt significant as in the story of *The Big and the Little Car and the Little Car Hiding*. I wondered if this reflected in some way his experience of relationships, not only the relationship we experienced in the therapy sessions but also other relationships, a child's relationship to a big world, an autistic child's relationship to the neurotypical world. On reflection, my conclusions on the processes at work are broader and I believe it was through a process of mutual attunement that we were able to work together. That unlocked the possibilities of adopting a developmental approach in the therapy and a pathway for impact and positive change. Through attunement, this vignette illustrates how a dramatherapy-informed approach can enable the therapeutic exploration of themes of relationship, communication, and nonverbal communication through the creation of a shared nonverbal narrative.

Attunement is a commonly used concept in the attachment literature. It has its roots in James' (1902/1982) theories of the 'unitive' feeling of connection with other people and life forms. Weber and Haen (2005) define attunement as 'the ability of caregivers and children to read each other's cues accurately, anticipate each other's needs and respond accordingly … through "tuning in" to cognitions, emotions, behaviours and physiology'. In *Building the Bonds of Attachment*, Hughes (2018, p. 7) describes how

> through attunement, the infant feels receptive to and connected to his parent and also can begin to regulate his affective states through first coregulating his affect to his parent's affective state. Through the addition of joint attention and intention, the infant can also begin to reflect on her inner life of thought, affect, and intentions, as well as the inner lives of her parents. She is able to co-create the meaning of the people, objects, and events of her life.

Attachment centres on the paradox that a safe-enough relationship, a secure base, allows the child to be alone in the company of the caregiver. The balance of dependence and autonomy permits the securely attached child to separate from the caregiver and explore the environment, operating from the knowledge that he can return physically or psychologically as needed for connection and co-regulation. Likewise, secure attachment relationships allow the dyad to engage flexibly with both positive and negative emotions.

In the attachment literature, attunement is often specified as affective attunement which Stern (1985, p. 142) has described as the 'performance of behaviours that express the quality of feeling cf a shared affect state without imitating the exact behavioural expression of the inner state'. Behaviour and responses related to emotion and relationships develop similarly through repeated mutual attunement within the dyad, which gradually leads to them being internalised in internal working models that are 'sensorimotor, procedural, and nonlinguistic in nature' (Mikulincer and Shaver, 2016).

It is linked to intersubjectivity, 'the infant's and parent's discovery of each other, and also the self in relation to the other' (Hughes, 2018). Hughes describes this experience of intersubjectivity as central to the development and coherence of the self and suggests that, while this is an early mother-child experience, it can be provided in a therapy setting. In therapy, he suggests that

the child experiences the impact she is having on the therapist (playfulness, acceptance, curiosity, and empathy) in response to any memory, experience or affective state, so that the child clarifies and deepens her subjective experience through the co-creation of meaning and welcomes the experience into the sense of self.

Therapy and the development of a therapeutic relationship offer opportunities for experiential and reparative attunement and attachment building. The process of attunement does not always proceed smoothly, so along with attunement comes mis-attunement and the need for repair. It is this potential for the repair of mis-attunement and repair through interaction that presents a therapeutic opportunity. The modes of delivery and communication of arts therapies are well suited to using this to positive effect (Kossak, 2009), particularly in nonverbal autistic young people; embodied action is a way forward (Weber and Haen, 2005). The essence of communication is generating a relationship where there is cooperation to make mutual meaning in a partnership with a dynamic feedback process (Bradshaw, 2001). This bidirectionality is of value when considering the place of arts therapy in working with nonverbal autistic people. Classical attachment theory and research have largely focused on the parental side of that relationship. An example is the Still Face Experiment (Mesman et al., 2009), first described in 1978; it focuses on the part played by the mother in creating communication and the effect that her withdrawal has on the child. It creates this focus especially in its presentation with a dominant narrator's voice. At the narrator's instruction, we are drawn to focus on the mother's role in the communication and the effect that her behaviour has on the child. We are not directed to look at the way the communication is co-constructed in the relationship with the child. Beatrice et al. (2010) have used microanalysis of mother-infant communication to identify the processes of communication, revealing the mother and infant as each influencing the other in a bi-directional, reciprocal, mutual regulation process.

These processes have relevance in two ways. First, the microanalysis identifies early pre-verbal communication between mother and infant as bi-directional, reciprocal, and mutually regulated. Second, the narrator's voice in the Still Face Experiment, as in other attachment theory, leads us to narrow our focus onto the role of the mother. The viewer identifies her as the main player because that is where we are directed to look. Attachment research has focused on the mother as the antecedent of infant attachment. Microanalysis of mother-infant communication places greater emphasis on the child's pattern of behaviour as well as the mother's, and considers the effect of these on the child and mother individually as well as interactively (Beebe and Steele, 2013). The implications of this for therapy with nonverbal autistic children is to confirm that, even from the earliest stages of development, communication is co-produced and bi-directional. This means that the child is always engaged and engageable in the creation of narrative in the facilitated creative interaction that is at the heart of all arts therapies.

In this case study, a narrative was created in the therapy session within the context of the therapeutic relationship. The relationship was built through the processes of attunement and bi-directional dyadic communication. In this way the communication paralleled processes of early communication and relationship-building using processes of observation and mirroring, or affect, attention and intention. Therapeutic intervention is not the same as parent-child attachment as it necessarily exists within the limited boundaries of therapy, but it seeks to build relationship and communication paralleling the dyadic parent-child experience. A broad construction of attunement means that the concept can be seen to include the relationship building and generation of a shared creative language that is fundamental to arts therapies.

---

**Case study 2: Sami's story – *Saving the Trains from the Underwater World***

*Sami had an Autism Spectrum Disorder diagnosis and was minimally verbal; he was a student at the resource base but had been almost fully integrated into the mainstream, we first met when he was aged 11. At the time we join him that integration had broken down and he had returned to the base. He was struggling to self-regulate and was often very distressed.*

*Being in control was important to Sami and helped him to avoid feeling overwhelmed. This behaviour may have been re-enforced by those around him as an understandable way of avoiding meltdowns. Sami had physical and verbal tics. The fact that he was compelled to produce involuntary sounds or movements added to his sense of being out of control. Sami used his language confidently but struggled to express his feelings. His language was idiosyncratic. When he was distressed, his language disintegrated into swearing and self-admonishment. Relationships were difficult for him and created stress. Other people were often a source of stress for Sami.*

*Sami used our dramatherapy sessions to create stories. All his stories were told through projective play using his favorite toys which were trains. This was a way of engaging and de-stressing. Sami seemed to like to come to the sessions and was usually pleased to see me. In the sessions, as well as witnessing his play, I had worked towards more mutual play first playing alongside him and later with him, inside the story. These offers were tolerated and accepted.*

*The week prior to this session Sami had been extremely distressed and dysregulated. He came to the session wearing ear defenders. In the session he created a story about an underwater world. The characters were terrified of drowning, of being overwhelmed by the water. In the session Sami had moments of quiet, they were not absences as I felt clear that he was present. I also noticed that he tasted the playdough he was using and that his vocal tics were present. He seemed to be processing the physical experience of the moment. In the story, the trains travelled through a portal into an underwater world. I offered blue material to be the water and Sami accepted it as part of his story. The trains were drowning! I offered a puppet to help but this was not accepted, instead, Sami made life jackets out of play dough for the trains. The trains were saved but the danger was not over as they were then attacked by crows! The crows were puppets. Sami named the puppets and expected me to operate them which I did.*

*The session had a dreamlike quality. After the session, I realised the story was a repeat from two weeks before where characters were overwhelmed in the underwater world. I wondered about the fact that Sami had returned to a story he had told before the period of dysregulation as well as the dreamlike quality of the session. Sami seemed to be using the repeated themes of the story to restore order and return to a state where he felt regulated.*

## Analysis

There is much to be gained by interdisciplinary working founded on a respectful understanding of the approaches of other professional groups. Sami worked with me as a dramatherapist and also with a Speech and Language Therapist (SLT). Speech and Language Therapy is not an arts therapy, but its theory and practice draw on the understandings of attachment theory, emotional regulation and theories of play that are fundamental to arts therapies. As part of therapy and in preparing this chapter, I discussed Sami with the SLT working with him. She framed her intervention in terms of SCERTS and *Intensive Interaction*. SCERTS (Social Communication Emotional Regulation and Transactional Support; Prizant et al., 2006) is an assessment and communication system which is developmentally sequenced into three levels of partnership: social, language, and communication. Sami was working between the second and third levels and the aim at this stage was to develop his interest and wonder in the social world and his desire to communicate. *Intensive Interaction* is an approach (Hewett et al., 1998) to develop reciprocal play, it aims to build the fundamentals of communication and show the child that communication is worthwhile, fun and reciprocal. The first step is for the child to notice the other person and to re-cognise that they are there. The therapist can then gradually add in offers for the child to follow and will follow offers made by the child. In this way the child begins to become aware that they can direct the play and that the therapist will follow them. Over time this process may build to more reciprocal play where offers are made and accepted on both sides.

In this second case study, reflecting on our experience of working with the same child in dramatherapy, we recognised similar aims (reciprocal play, social interaction, emotional regulation, and agency) but the way we met these had differences. Like dramatherapy, SLT draws on psychodynamic processes and attachment theory; unlike dramatherapy, the SLT's role is more consistent with the concept of Vygotsky's *More Knowledgeable Other* (1978) where primary importance is placed on social interaction and the co-construction of knowl-edge in partnership with guidance from that More Knowledgeable Other. While Vygotsky's work has informed arts therapy theory, in dramatherapy, the focus is more on the experience of attunement (as discussed above) and agency. In dramatherapy, we might use scaffolding to support the child in their rela-tionship building, but the ownership of the narrative belongs to the child and the role of the therapist is to support the child in what they wish to express. It is of interest that different stances of the position of the therapist in relation to the client did not seem to affect the extent to which there was success in achieving these aims. Indeed, the synergy and discussion with the SLT was of value not only in informing my own understanding and practice of dramatherapy, but also in enhancing the overall therapeutic outcome.

---

**Case study 3: Twinkle's story – *Jack Gets No Game***

*The sessions were with a girl with a ten-year-old diagnosis of Autism Spectrum Disorder and selective mutism. Twinkle is not her name but the name her parent asked me to use in this vignette when we discussed consent. As a part of a period of assessment I offered Twinkle a six-part story structure (Lahad, 1992). Twinkle created a story through images and written words. The story was about a boy called Jack who wanted a Nintendo game. He was told that he could have the game but only if he did his chores. Jack did not have the money to buy the game himself and did not want to do the chores, so he decided to get other people to do his chores. He asked a lot of people but they all said 'no!' At the end of the story, the chores were not done and Jack did not get his game. The story was called Jack Gets No Game.*

## Analysis

As discussed above, there is considerable heterogeneity in the aetiology of nonverbalism in autistic children. Twinkle had selective mutism as well as being autistic. Selective mutism is a severe anxiety disorder where a person is unable to speak in certain social situations, such as with classmates at school or relatives they do not see very often. A child or adult with selective mutism does not refuse or choose not to speak at certain times, they are literally unable to speak. The expectation to talk to certain people triggers a freeze response with feelings of panic and talking is impossible. It affects 1 in 140 people and is more common in girls. Autistic people have high comorbidity with anxiety and other mental disorders as well as with learning disabilities; so, as with Twinkle, autism and selective mutism can co-exist. Given the different aetiology, it is of interest to see how therapeutic approaches may differ.

Storymaking is central to dramatherapy as a way to communicate, through distanced metaphor, aspects of the client's internal world or lived experience. In Twinkle's story it was striking that Jack could have got the game if he had just done his chores, but instead he refused and chose to ask others. In this way, the story revolved around a refusal. Jack had no money. His parent said 'no' to buying him the game unless he did his chores. Jack said 'no' to this and asked others to do his chores. They all said 'no', so Jack had no game. There were 11 'no's in the short story; a cycle of 'no!'.

The story was fascinating in the light of Twinkle's selective mutism; her own silent 'no'. With this child I often found myself reliant on words. When I reflect, I can see that I was pushing a verbal agenda when none was offered. In contrast, Twinkle often expressed a desire to move and be free in the space. In terms of attunement the story helps us, but my instinctive flight to verbalism perhaps did not. To explore this case study further I met with a Play Therapist who also had experience of working with autistic children with selective mutism.

In her work, the therapist described 'narrating aloud' what she saw and 'reflecting through wonderings'. The Play Therapist's view was that the child's authorship of the stories created in play was held within the play with the therapist's 'wonderings' reflecting that play. Sometimes children offered their own verbal narrative alongside the play. However, as this was not possible in a case of selective mutism, the therapist offered her own 'loose injection of wondering', and the child wrote messages in the therapy. The therapist named that, in her work with autistic children, she observed that the stories created in play were always rooted in reality. She illustrated this with an example in which a child created play adventures using characters from a cartoon played by the therapist and the child. In the session, the therapist and the child went on adventures created by the child as these characters. My understanding of this is that the child transposed characters that represented the relationship that had been created with the therapist in the therapy sessions and then created stories/adventures. The Play Therapist saw this as based in reality, whereas I saw the use of the characters as a language to describe the therapeutic relationship as experienced in the sessions which was then repositioned into imaginative play. These interpretive differences notwithstanding, we both agreed that the key to developing and using communication in the therapy was enabling progressive attunement, and that while this was true in all therapy sessions it was especially so in work with nonverbal or minimally verbal clients where communication was experienced primarily somatically and through attunement.

## Discussion

In this chapter, I have argued for the therapeutic value of arts therapies in the support of nonverbal and minimally verbal autistic children. I identify that the ability of arts and non-arts therapies, in their different ways, to enable meaningful attunement is a shared keystone in their effectiveness and therefore of fundamental importance. In all arts therapies, there is a focus on attunement with the client. In dramatherapy, this is achieved through the co-creation of a narrative using imagination, therapeutic alliance, metaphor, play and a language of expression that works for the client.

What all arts therapies have in common is an understanding of attachment, early experiences, and relationship building. The use of arts modalities to enable attunement to allow the development of new ways of communicating through therapy, and to repair mis-attunement where that has occurred using the fundamental developmental processes, is of no less importance in nonverbal autistic children than in their neurotypical peers. Arts therapies are by design fundamentally inclusive and welcoming to those that are different and have expressive difficulties. The flexibility, accessibility and nonverbal nature of the practice of arts therapies makes them particularly accessible and attractive to those with autism and learning disabilities, and to those who are nonverbal or minimally verbal. Arts therapies deliver the kind of attunement that is seen in effective psychotherapy characterised by a balanced level of predictability that is neither overly stable nor too erratic (Beebe et al., 2016).

From Beebe's critique of the Still Face Experiment (Beebe et al., 2016), we see that even at the earliest phases of communication, there is bidirectionality in communication. Arts therapies all recognise that this is the case, even if the client is not neurotypical or verbal. They recognise that the therapeutic relationship is built on both sides through detailed observation and attunement. When considering autism, the move from a restrictive hierarchy of low to the high ability to a constellation of different strengths and difficulties is very much in line with the eclectic and personally tailored approaches taken by arts therapists. The words of Naoki Higashida (2013) in *The Reason Why I Jump* are an eloquent reminder that a lack of speech does not equate with a lack of thought. Simple constructions of nonverbalism in autism as a direct function of learning disability and consequent therapeutic nihilism are no longer tenable. Arts therapies can and do help.

## Conclusion

The case studies and discussion in this chapter are supportive of arts therapies in the care of nonverbal autistic children. Its support for therapeutic intervention goes wider with the positive inclusion of Speech and Language Therapy and Play Therapy. The common denominator is attunement; the fundamental value of attunement applies not only to therapists but to all clinicians in their interactions with their clients. Bradley Peterson (2019), the director of the Institute for the Developing Mind at San Francisco Children's Hospital, in his analysis of the art of healing concludes, 'shared understanding, interpersonal attunement, and alliance between clinicians and their patients ... together constitute the true science and art of healing'. We need to find ways of listening to those who cannot speak, and arts therapies provide a way to hear the nonverbal autistic child. Their practice enables both parts of the therapeutic dyad to find a language to listen; attunement is the bidirectional process by which we listen, learn, and change through therapy.

## Note

1   The name and details of the cases in this chapter have been modified to preserve anonymity in accordance with the consent obtained.

## References

Baio, J., Wiggins, L., Christensen, D.L., Maenner, M.J., Daniels, J., Warren, Z., et al. (2018) 'Prevalence of autism spectrum disorder among children aged 8 years – Autism and developmental disabilities monitoring network, 11 Sites, United States, 2014', *Morbidity and Mortality Weekly Report. Surveillance Summaries*, 67(6), pp. 1–23. 10.15585/mmwr.ss6706a1

Beatrice, B., Joseph, J., Markese, S., Buck, K., Chen, H., Cohen, P., Bahrick, L., Andrews, H. and Feldstein, S. (2010) 'The origins of 12-month attachment: A microanalysis of 4-month mother–infant interaction', *Attachment & Human Development*, 12(1–2), pp. 3–141, doi: 10.1080/14616730903338985.

Beebe, B. and Steele, M. (2013) 'How does microanalysis of mother-infant communication inform maternal sensitivity and infant attachment?' *Attachment & Human Development*, 15(5–6), pp. 583–602. 10.1080/14616734.2013.841050.

Beebe, B., Messinger, D., Bahrick, L.E., Margolis, A., Buck, K.A. and Chen, H. (2016) 'A systems view of mother-infant face-to-face communication', *Developmental Psychology*, 52(4), pp. 556–571. 10.1037/a0040085.

Bradshaw J. (2001) Communication partnerships with people with profound and multiple learning disabilities.*Tizard Learning Disability Review*, 6, pp. 6–15.

Danon-Boileau L. (2001) *The silent child exploring the world of children who do not speak*. Oxford: Oxford University Press.

Fletcher-Watson S. and Happe, S. (2018) *Autism: A new introduction to psychological theory and current debate*. 2nd edn. London: Routledge.

Gardener, H. (1983) *Frames of mind: The theory of multiple intelligences*. New York City: Basic Books.

Hewett, D. and Nind, M. (1998) *Interaction in action: Reflections on the use of intensive interaction*. London: David Fulton Publishers.

Higashida, N. (2013) *The reason I jump: The inner voice of a thirteen-year-old boy with autism*. First edition. New York: Random House.

Hughes, D. (2018). *Building the bonds of attachment*. Third edition. London: Roman & Littlefield.

Interagency Autism Coordinating Committee (2011). *IACC strategic plan for autism spectrum disorder research*. Washington, D.C.: Department of Health and Human Services. Accessed 13 June 2021 https://iacc.hhs.gov/publications/strategic-plan/2011/.

James, W. (1902/1958) *The varieties of religious experience*. New York: The New American Library, Inc.

Kossak, M.S. (2009) 'Therapeutic attunement: A transpersonal view of expressive arts therapy', *The Arts in Psychotherapy*, 36, pp. 13–18.

Lahad, M. (1992) Storymaking in assessment method for coping with stress', in S. Jennings (ed.) *Dramatherapy theory and practice II*. London: Routledge, pp. 150–163.

Mesman, J., van Ijzendoorn, M.H. and Bakermans-Kranenburg, M.J. (2009) 'The many faces of the still-face paradigm: A review and meta-analysis', *Developmental Review*, 29(2), pp. 120–162.

Munson, J., Dawson, G., Sterling, L., Beauchaine, T., Zhou, A., Kohler, E., et al. (2008) 'Evidence for latent classes of IQ in young children with autism spectrum disorder', *American Journal on Mental Retardation*, 113, pp. 438–452.

Mikulincer, M. and Shaver, P.R. (2016) *Attachment in adulthood: Structure, dynamics, and change*, 2nd ed., New York: Guilford.

Peterson, B.S. (2019) 'Editorial: Common factors in the art of healing', *Journal of Child Psychology Psychiatry*, 60, pp. 927–929. 10.1111/jcpp.13108.

Prizant, B.M., Wetherby, A.M., Rubin, E., Laurent, A.C. and Rydell, P. (2006) *The SCERTS model: A comprehensive educational approach for children with autism spectrum disorders*. Baltimore: Paul H. Brookes Publishing.

Rapin, I., Dunn, M., Allen, D., Stevens, M. and Fein, D. (2009) 'Subtypes of language disorders in school-age children with autism', *Developmental Neuropsychology*, 34, pp. 66–84.

Stern, D.N. (1985) *The interpersonal world of the infant*. New York: Basic Books.

Tager-Flusberg, H. and Kasari, C. (2013) 'Minimally verbal school-aged children with autism spectrum disorder: the neglected end of the spectrum', *Autism Research: Official Journal of the International Society for Autism Research*, 6(6), pp. 468–478. /10.1002/aur.1329.

Tager-Flusberg, H., Paul, R. and Lord, C.E. (2005) 'Language and communication in autism', in F. Volkmar, R. Paul, A. Klin and D.J. Cohen (eds.) *Handbook of autism and pervasive developmental disorder*. 3. Vol. 1. New York: Wiley.

Vygotsky, L.S. (1978) *Mind in society: The development of higher psychological processes*. Massachusetts: Harvard University Press.

Weber, A.M. and Haen, C. (2005) 'Attachment-informed drama therapy with adolescents' in S. Jennings and C. Holmwood (eds.) *Routledge international handbook of dramatherapy*. London: Routledge.

Widdowson, M. (2011) 'Case study research methodology', *International Journal of Transactional Analysis Research & Practice*, 2(1), pp. 25–34. 10.29044/v2i1p25.

Chapter 14

# "The Art of Receiving"

A Heuristic Narrative Exploration of Long-Term Art Therapy with a Young Person with Autism from the Perspectives of Therapist, Client and Parent

*Nicki Power, with collaborative input from Roger Arguile, Marshall Bourne, and Kerry Bourne*

## Introduction

This chapter chronicles the 'tacit knowing' (Polanyi, 1967) shared from the different perspectives of an art therapist, client and parent, who had all been part of a six-year individual art therapy journey. Each told the story of art therapy from their point of view to Nicki, an invited witness. The words written here are drawn from two encounters. One between Nicki and Roger, both art therapists and the second between Nicki, Marshall, the client, and Kerry, his Mum. Writing this chapter represents a flickering still from a film reel: a snapshot of the complex and multi-layered experiences shared between Roger, Marshall and Kerry during art therapy and in the intervening years.

Roger and Marshall met for weekly individual art therapy when Marshall was in school in England, beginning when he was aged 12. Roger also used his therapeutic skills to offer staff in the school a different way of seeing Marshall. In parallel with the confidential creative space that he offered Marshall, Roger supported Kerry along the journey, validating Kerry's awareness of Marshall's many strengths and also modelling clear boundaries to transfer the changes made in art therapy to their home. In 2019, with Marshall due to leave school for college and Roger set to retire, their art therapy ended. Also in that year, though not whilst he was working with Marshall, Roger received a devastating diagnosis of motor neuron disease.

Our impetus to write this chapter began with two aims. First Roger wanted to share: *"anything that … might be of a little help to someone, you know, might resonate with someone about something of use"*. Here, he refers modestly to his 40 years of clinical practice as an art therapist and the wealth of knowledge he holds about working with young people with autism. The second aim was to include Marshall and Kerry, not as

DOI: 10.4324/9781003201656-18

anonymised or de-identified participants, but as vibrant people with equally valid experiences to share within this partnership.

In the summer of 2022, I, Nicki, the author of this chapter, travelled to Berkshire, in the South-East of England, to meet a stranger in his home. This was my first encounter with Roger. That day Marshall and Kerry were unable to travel from Kent to join us. Several weeks later, technology failed us, and we could not meet online, though we did catch vivid and jittery video images of each other in our own homes. A phone-call on loudspeaker meant that Marshall and Kerry could still share their stories with Nicki. Roger died in October 2022, just as we were finalising this chapter.

## Study Approach

### Theoretical Position

Our theoretical position is grounded in social constructivism, viewed through the lens of critical disability. This means that our knowledge and understanding is created in our social world. Specifically, when we think about disability, which may be how the diagnosis of autism is viewed, we see it as a socially constructed issue, not a problem which is located within a person. The same position has informed the philosophical underpinnings of the research methodology used. The overall narrative approach we have adopted is also rooted in social constructionism; this allowed for the different stories to unfold presenting multiple perspectives constructed by the therapists, the participant and his parent.

### Defining Roles and Collaborative Working

We approached this chapter collaboratively, recognising that each person had a unique contribution to make to the process. As a group, we negotiated the roles we would take. Roger, Marshall and Kerry did not want to write, but wanted to share their experiences with me, Nicki; I took the lead in writing the chapter. We agreed that they would review the draft chapter and changes were then made.

Deciding on authorship was the most challenging part of our collaboration for me. I had hoped that we would be co-authors, based on my past experience of the ways in which different people can contribute to academic knowledge (Power et al., 2022), and thus share power in the process. However, Roger felt strongly that I should be the sole author. In a telephone call, he described my role as: "*voyeuristic. You are looking, you are an artist. In looking you're receiving the accuracy of what happened. That's good*". This perspective supported me to see that my own socio-cultural lens coloured the writing. Regardless of the care taken during the collaborative process, I would never write a chapter as Roger or Marshall or Kerry might, and that was okay.

Throughout the chapter, the words of each person are shown in italics with quotations. Following the narrative research tradition, I wanted to keep the voices of Roger, Marshall and Kerry at the core of this work, since it could not have been written without their rich contributions.

### Ethical Considerations

Each person voluntarily agreed to take part in the process of making this chapter. We were not aligned to a particular organisation and so did not seek institutional ethical approval. We were guided by the RESPECT Code of Practice (2004). This is a voluntary pan-European framework which supports independent practitioners to conduct research ethically and professionally. Some of our ethical considerations were:

- Providing an accessible means for all collaborators to contribute meaningfully, through meeting in person, online or by telephone.
- Negotiating the level of involvement each person wanted in developing the chapter.
- Ensuring a review mechanism once the chapter was written, both for sense-checking and to maintain a sense of safety, given the personal nature of this method.
- Engaging with each other, along with our editors and trusted peers, to support fully informed decision making where changes were considered.

### Methods

Whilst there is a broad spectrum of narrative approaches in research, this narrative inquiry is grounded in personal storytelling, explored "in communicative relation" (Gubrium and Holstein, 2008, p. 243), which enabled knowledge of wider social phenomena to be revealed. The lived experiences were shared verbally; however, stories were also embodied, told within a relational and temporal context (Hydén and Antelius, 2011). This led to a co-constructed narrative exploration, grounded in the relational interplay between the collaborators and I.

When using qualitative methods, the researcher is part of the phenomenon under investigation and will be affected by it. I adopted an heuristic lens (Moore, 2020) which incorporated my lived experience as an art therapist working with people with autism as a core component of the investigation. The heuristic method does not seek objective detachment; instead it favours a systematic but fluid inquiry process (Douglass and Moustakas, 1985) which privileges personal engagement and reflexivity by the researcher to enhance meaning making (Moustakas, 1990).

Typically, the phases of both narrative and heuristic inquiry are not linear; they may be cyclical and usually occur in parallel, so cannot be described as distinct phases of the research. A combination of narrative and arts-based methods were used to explore the experiences shared, to discover meaning and to extend accessibility (Hydén and Antelius, 2011; Nyman, Josephsson and Isaksson, 2012). Furthermore, due to the iterative nature of the process, both data collection and analysis occurred in parallel. This mixed-qualitative methodology allowed for complex life experiences which hold a particular meaning for the participants to be shared and considered, so that similarities and differences emerge, before a cohesive understanding can be reached.

I used unstructured interviews to explore the meaning and experience of art therapy for the other collaborators. I met with Roger in person for two and a half hours and I met separately with Marshall and Kerry for a further hour, speaking by telephone. I recorded the meetings and transcribed these. From 3.5 hours in each other's lives I had:

- 40 pages of transcribed discussion
- Borrowed copies of two hard-backed books filled with glorious, coloured photos of artwork which Roger had made - one of Marshall's art and one of his own
- Photos taken on the visit to Roger's home.

After the meetings, we kept in touch through phone calls, emails and text messages. I also amassed scribbled fragments of poetry written in snatched moments following both encounters and in the intervening weeks.

While immersed in the data, through listening to the voice recordings and transcribing them, I noticed the gentle tinkling of softly played music which was the backdrop to my encounter with Roger. I then read and re-read the printed transcripts, using a felt-tip marker to highlight each line or phrase that resonated. Each line was then transferred to a post-it note, linked by a page number back to the original transcript, and I began to sort and organise the data segments into themes. This became the frame for the chapter, which was given life as Roger's, Marshall's and Kerry's words were woven together by me. The process of consolidating the meaning was through further discussion with Roger primarily, but also with Marshall and Kerry. Further moments of meaning were identified, and I could amend our narrative by redrafting the chapter.

Finally, my use of poetry acted as the creative synthesis (Moustakas, 1990) which completed the heuristic narrative approach to this study. Borrowing Furman's (2020) approach to poetic inquiry as radical data compression I used both found lines in the transcripts and my own poetic response to create a series of poems in response to this work, one of which is included in this chapter.

This whole experience was quite compressed, occurring within a three-month period in 2022.

## Parts of a Story

The following sections weave together the experiences shared by Roger, Marshall and Kerry from my perspective. We begin with a close-up shot, sharing Marshall's story of individual art therapy, then the camera pans out to include both Roger's and Kerry's experiences. Next, we take a step back, a wide-angle shot, to see how art therapy might help other children and young people with autism. Finally, we return to the immediacy of these intimate encounters as I experienced them.

Roger, Marshall and Kerry are reflecting on six years of weekly, individual art therapy, which Marshall attended, beginning when he was 12 years old and attended a school for children with special educational needs. Roger did not have motor neuron disease when they worked together. They also discuss what has happened since art therapy ended and how their relationships have changed.

### (Part of) Marshall's Story

In school, Marshall was referred to see Roger for art therapy "*because of his appalling behaviour*". Roger described him "*as a whirlwind*" saying "*he was so naughty and so wonderful*". From the start of their relationship, Roger saw more in Marshall than a child who "*exploded*" by shouting and breaking objects. Marshall recalled that "*my anger and my depressed situation*" were what brought him to art therapy. Kerry stated that before art therapy Marshall "*was very frowny*". Marshall agreed and added: "*frowny and confused*". Kerry said: "*You didn't know how to be, because of your autism*". Marshall gave the example of how he used to: "*disrupt class or assembly and just wasting it*".

When I talked with Marshall, about what he remembered of being in art therapy, in those early days, he said: "*With Roger we talk together and it's like such a useful thing we do … we did have some [eye] contact, you know, but usually, I stare at the paper and that's just great. He understood I may not have the best eye contact*". In his understated way, Roger recalled: "*And we'd just sit together, I'd watch him. He'd be next to me and I'd watch him. We'd chat a bit. [pause] We'd laugh a bit*". This was Roger attuning to Marshall's needs in the art therapy sessions.

Roger described the psychological process that he believed was occurring in his relationship with Marshall, through art therapy. He said, children with autism:

> don't know about what the other person is going to do or think or say. It's fear, fear of the unknown. … This fear autistic children have, of being invaded, means they cannot receive. And what it means to receive is to open your heart in some way. That's terrifying to the autistic person.

When speaking about starting art therapy with children, just like Marshall he said:

> I would work with them as if they were very frightened animals ... almost primitive senses, like an animal. I don't mean that in a derogatory way. ... They're so attuned to sound and movement ... it's good for the therapist also to be attuned to those things. And not just be there thinking I'll interpret this picture.

Kerry had great insight into the process of art therapy as she thought it might have played out for Marshall:

> I could imagine him with Roger being really ... tense, but then it's just a way of letting yourself go ... it helped him to be able to do something else with his hands and express himself with the drawing. And then it's like how he was feeling then flowed from his mouth because he was relaxed.

Slowly, over time, meeting week in and week out, in this art therapy dyad, *"things that had been a threat, stopped being a threat ... he felt safe ... he was able to receive"*. Roger believed that Marshall *"realised he was a person that could be liked and valued and heard and listened to. ... I think it took therapy ... for him to be able to receive that"*.

Marshall spoke about his choice of art materials: *"most common consists with pencil, sketching and sometimes with pens too. And ... ink drawing"*. Largely, the subject matter he drew consisted of: *"a lot of buildings ... things with straight lines and ruler"*. I thought this was an understatement too, as I'd seen the hard-backed book Roger had made for Marshall of his art. It contained detailed cityscapes and landscapes full of activity and inhabitants. There were technical drawings of machines and systems that reminded me of Da Vinci's complex plans for yet-to-be-invented objects. The image that Marshall picked (Figure 14.1) to be included in this chapter doesn't have a name. It has the words *"Live in Colour"* written on it and is one of the few drawings that has coloured elements, supplementing his monochromatic line drawings. He said: *"I've done that. I didn't give it a title. I think it's [a] symbolic story ... You can always look at other things, be more expressive"*.

Alongside working with Marshall, Roger described working with other members of Marshall's support network: staff in the school and Kerry. He recalled wistfully that Marshall:

> used to go out at playtime and throw water in puddles up in the air, or on a dry day throw dust high in the air and watch it fall. Which is exactly like the land artist, Andy Goldsworthy, would, but because he's autistic and at school, staff would say: *"Oh, Marshall, don't do that. You're gonna get so*

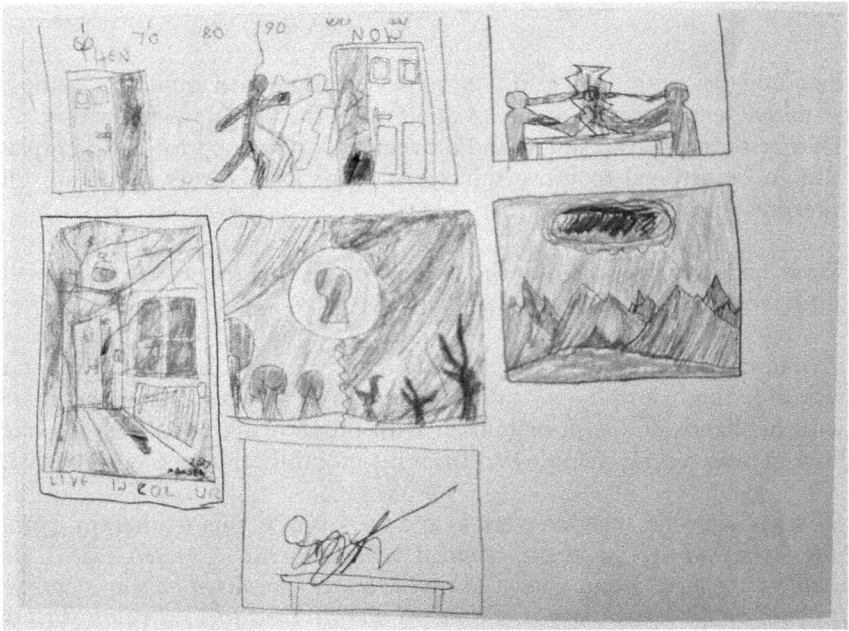

*Figure 14.1* Photograph of untitled artwork made by Marshall in art therapy from "Marshall's Drawings", a book prepared by Roger Arguille

*dirty*". So I'd talk to staff a little bit and say: "*yes he is and it's a bit of a drag, but he's a mad scientist and [a] mad artist thrown into one. He's doing some interesting things. I should let him do that*".

Here, there's an ease in how Roger describes allaying the anxieties of staff members while simultaneously validating Marshall's experimental playfulness. While this is not direct therapeutic work within the confines of the art therapy studio with Marshall, this holistic engagement with Marshall's support network was an essential part of supporting Marshall to be understood outside of art therapy.

The changes which Marshall attributed to art therapy began as "*helping getting ready [for] when I'm back into class. It's like a way to cope with the struggles and difficulties of preparing to [go] to another class*". He also talked about art therapy helping him to "*stop being too shy and talked a lot [more]*". The ripples of change seen in school, also reached his home life, as we'll see when Kerry shared her story, and they filtered through to his internal world. Both Marshall and Kerry made a link between the work in art therapy and how it has supported Marshall to grow into the "*adult he wants to be*". Kerry believes that "*we wouldn't have the Marshall we've got now, who's quite understanding*" *and able to express himself".* And Marshall thought: *"I'd be the other way round … I would have been the same negative guy"* without art therapy.

### (Part of) Kerry's Story

Kerry spoke about the power of the label of autism and the fear it can bring: *"when you find out your child has a disability … you get told negatives from day one … as a parent of a child with autism, you can get worried … because you don't know what to do".* When Marshall was diagnosed, there was little support for family members or carers of children with autism; she said: *"we felt quite isolated".* She spoke about the importance of relationship building, by professionals with parents, to ensure the child receives the right help: *"you can always get the vibe of the ones that actually care. And you're not just a person, like a number, like a job".*

Taking his therapeutic work beyond the art therapy studio, Roger visited the family at home on two occasions to work with them when, as Kerry put it: *"Marshall was quite angry at home … and a little bit thinking he was in charge".* Roger recalled saying to Marshall:

> when you come in at the end of the day, Marshall, you kick the door. Is that right? And he said *"Yes I do, yea"* and I said well if you go [Roger makes a loud knocking sound with his fist on the table] that's a better idea. *"Oh, oh yea, oh yes okay".* So I think he respected me.

Interestingly, all three agreed that Marshall changed from kicking the door when he got home to knocking on it, because he respected Roger. The word respect was used several times in each encounter. I felt a strong sense of mutual respect between Roger, Marshall and Kerry.

What Kerry observed was that Roger *"set the same kind of boundaries at home … and it helped Marshall understand how to behave at school and at home".* She was then able to put this into practice herself. Roger said, by phone: *"in my territory [the art therapy studio] he felt safe, then in his territory he was able to receive what I said there because of the art therapy".* Kerry talked about learning *"to stay a lot calmer, because I've heard the way Roger speaks".* She also noticed that Roger broke information down in a *"step by step sort of way".* Later we spoke about how Roger modelled how to *"talk to him age appropriate,"* regardless of autism being there or not, whilst making sure to *"explain things a little bit more".* As she spoke, I felt a sense of her empowerment as a Mum, knowing how to support Marshall, and feeling more supported herself.

Kerry spoke about how working alongside Roger had changed her too: *"he just taught me to have a more positive outlook on Marshall's future".* She made a link between both Marshall and Roger being artists and how this helped build her own confidence and validate her understanding of

Marshall's strengths: *"Having someone who is an artist as well ... and he thinks Marshall's awesome. ... My boy is awesome, you know? ... Just having another person to champion your child is nice because you don't get that often"*.

After we met, Kerry sent me a photograph of Roger and Marshall (Figure 14.2) which she had taken when they visited Roger at his studio after art therapy had ended (discussed later in this chapter). She said it is her favourite photograph of them together.

### (Part of) Roger's Story

When I met Roger, we did not start by exploring Marshall's story. He introduced his life as an artist and later an art therapist to me, through two hard-backed books he had made, containing his work. These were: *"Raw Material"* and *"Art.Therapy"*. They were collections of his vast body of artistic output, neatly contained within bound edges. Much of his work used mixed-media, often made through a combination of portraits captured in

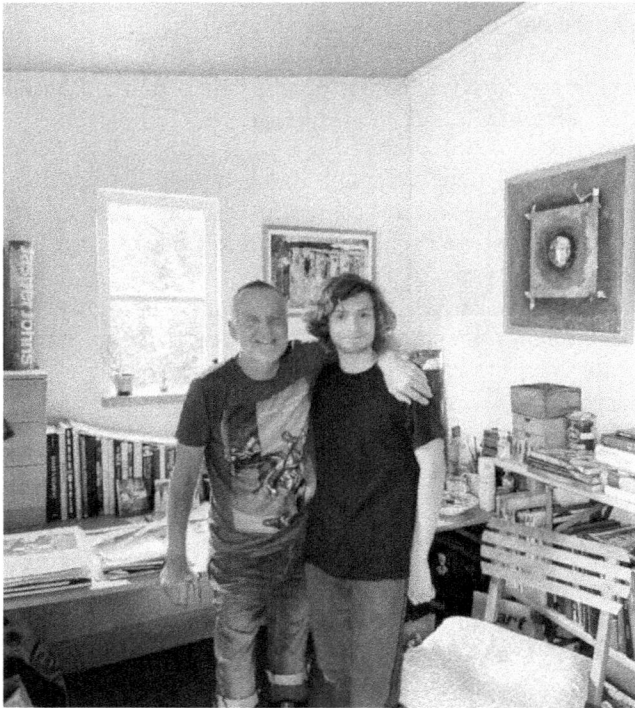

*Figure 14.2* Photograph of Roger and Marshall in Roger's Studio in 2020, taken by Kerry

photographs (of people both known and unknown), found objects and painting. Scherly (2015) interviewed Roger at a solo exhibition he held, and she said of his work:

> The guiding thread of the work seems to be people, portraits or fleeting shots in motion, all, or nearly, anonymous. My gut was speaking a nameless language but one thing was for sure, I *really* looked and I could *really* feel.

Roger was inspired by cinema. He said: "*I've always been interested in the flickering lights that film conjures up, evocative images of your family or whatever*". This he attributed to his grandfather's cataloguing of family events through the use of "*super 8*" film. He spoke both of "*the passage of time*" in films and the potential through "*freeze-framing the images*" to capture moments that could be "*frozen in an image*". Thus, the portraits emerged from moving-pictures.

When Scherly (2015) asked about his motivation, he said it was: "about honouring or preserving in some rather respectful way the image of some person". To me he said: "*it's always been about looking back at the beauty … and the innocence of being*". And so Roger picked as the piece of artwork he would like to be included, a found photograph he had worked on (Figure 14.3); captured as a photograph within his book, "*Raw Material*".

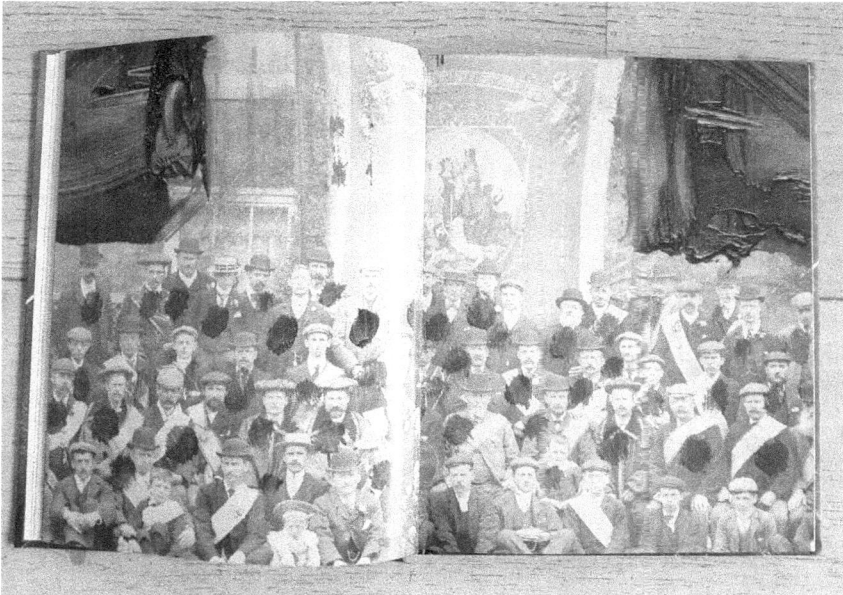

*Figure 14.3* Photograph of mixed-media image from "Raw Material" by Roger Arguile

He said about this artwork, that "*a photograph is like touch, like connection,*" you can feel something of the people captured for that moment in time. This is a photograph he bought at Bexhill-on-Sea. He doesn't know the men in the image. He used "*rather blood-like oil paint*" and "*kind of marked everyone's life*". Referring to his process, he said: "*I marked one, thought, I can't leave the others out. I wanted to honour them. To honour their existence*".

There was a third book, one which I did not see the pages of. It was a black-covered sketchbook placed within Roger's reach, where he currently makes art. He said: "*it's the first time ever, I would consider my work as therapeutically valuable to me*". Now, living with motor neuron disease his art-making process has had to adapt.

My most recent work is on A4 paper with a biro ... which I hold in a funny way because my fingers are folding in, because of the motor neuron disease, and I've been doing a lot of drawings, sort of me really. Very, very personal really. About how I'm coping with this disease.

### Revealing the Elements of Art Therapy Practice with Young People with Autism

The last hard-backed book that Roger shared with me was *Marking Time*. A portrait of his art therapy practice with young people. This was the product of a video project in which he collaborated with his daughter Rachel, also an art therapist. He revisited six children who had autism, years after their art therapy had ended, and talked with them about their memory of art therapy while Rachel recorded film and took photos (Arguile, 2012). As we talked, Roger used the word "*reveal*" and I added "*the meaning in the work ... the difference it can make and the core of what art therapy actually does*". This was the point when we both realised that we were exploring fundamental elements of art therapy practice that support children with autism to find meaning and to make changes.

For Roger, building relationships was central to his work: "*for autistic people in therapy, you know, it was still about making the relationship*". He expanded on this, defining a key task for the art therapist as: "*to find the place where the potential for communication is, and go there*". This mirrors Schweizer, Knorth and Spreens' (2014) findings in their systematic review that "art is another language to share experiences. Art therapy is described as an alternative way of communicating, because art stands between the child and the therapist" (2014, p. 589). One way to do this, which Roger used, was: "*working with their interest is often the thing*". He suggested using curiosity to 'meet the person where they're at' in order to begin to lay the foundations of trust.

Roger also focussed on sensory aspects of the work. He described children who were "*very attuned to their senses ... to sound and movement*". Martin

(2009) in her viewpoint paper agrees that sensory regulation in art therapy with children with autism "is often less stressful ... because the art provides a product to focus on beyond the process of integrating uncomfortable sensory experiences" (2009, p. 188). The process of art making becomes a safe way to transform sensory information and begin to process experiences.

Beginning in 1985, Roger grew his clinical art therapy practice within a school setting, supporting young people with special educational needs, which often included children with autism. Roger has described some elements of his art therapy practice in other publications (Case and Dalley, 1990, 1992). He is a competent writer, with a clear theoretical position, firmly grounded in art-based practice (Waller & Gilroy, 1992). When he describes case material, he consistently does this in a non-stigmatising and non-pathologising way. All of this, I learned after our meeting, flicking through art therapy books I'd owned for years, but in which I'd never noticed Roger's name. I was able to re-visit his printed words with new eyes.

When working with Marshall, Roger had spoken about "*being able to receive*" as moving beyond relational transactions ("*how to give and how to take*"), and away from "*psychological threat*" to a personal sense of being "*good enough*" (Winnicott, 1971). This is also linked to the therapist's "*unconditional positive regard*" (Rogers, 1957, p. 96) in that "*through therapy, to receive, not just know it, but receive the fact that [the client is] liked*" for who they are, just as they are. For the client to reach the point of "*being able to receive*," Roger considered some of the tasks required of the therapist are:

- To provide "*accurate empathy*": a titrated emotional response which ensures "*the child [is] receiving the right sort of help*" linked to the aims of their art therapy.
- To introduce "*safe confrontation*": an inter-personal challenge which ensures that "*the client can receive that as a helpful thing not as a criticism*" so that growth is possible.
- To be a "*helpful disruptor*" in challenging a person's thoughts, habits or repetition (in behaviour or artmaking). This break in behaviour gives the potential for something new to occur in art therapy, which can later be translated to other areas of life.

Roger also discussed the importance of being an embodied artist. While Roger chose not to make art alongside the children he worked with, he embodied the role of an artist. His paintings in progress were always on view in the art therapy studio. We both agreed that: "*you've got to be an artist who understands the language of art and the power of that language*". He spoke of how important it is that "*therapists use what they find interesting, and it's very important that therapists let themselves be interested and not sort of, push away or apologise for being interested. ... You just can't sit there*". Being open as a therapist is linked to uncertainty, above, but perhaps more directly to the authenticity of the art therapist: "*Because no matter what you do, if you're a therapist you are in the session*". For Roger, this meant being in a studio and "*showing*" his artist identity, not having the answers but being able to wonder with the client about what could be possible. This authenticity enables connection between the therapist and the client "*on a human level*".

Woven throughout these elements of art therapy practice were creativity and confidence. Roger understood that, as Winnicott said, "*psychotherapy has to do with two people playing together*" (1971, p. 51) and this requires both experimentation and adaptation. Furthermore, that "*a sense of ease and confidence*" is needed, allowing the art therapist to adapt therapeutic boundaries, both flexing them creatively, perhaps by expanding to include working with parents, and re-stating the rules within the art studio that keep both the therapist and client safe.

### The Experience of Being and the Memory of Experience

During the narrative inquiry process, an additional motivation for writing this chapter emerged. Roger said: "*I feel I've got a few things to say still before I die, I'd quite like to have that in a recent form*". This frank honesty saturated our discussions. After reading the draft chapter, Roger said in a phone call: "*the emotional aspects of the disease have made the work I've done more poignant and more powerful now*". Kerry had said: "*I just want everyone to know him [Roger]*". After meeting all three, I too feel compelled to share not simply a successful art therapy case study but a touching story of human connection (Figure 14.4).

And sometimes the help is in the silence.
There it is between us. Some closeness.
Receiving gets easier through our alliance.

And sometimes the help is in the words.
They flowed from his mouth, now heard.
A wordless connection. He cares; he's there.

And sometimes the help comes in the making.
Two artists meeting. He understood. And I felt different.

*Figure 14.4* A triolet, written by Nicki, constructed from words found within the three interview transcripts

In art therapy, Roger "*hardly ever*" made art. At our meeting we did not make art together. Yet, this encounter for me was one of the most artistic and creative experiences I've had in my professional life. As we talked, the open-plan living space was filled with conversation about artists, from Rembrandt to Goldsworthy. Being with Roger, I felt in the presence of an artist. It's in his words and his understanding of the creative process; when we fail to translate the idea in our head to the canvas or when we debate internally what to add next to a mixed-media image and how, even now each piece added still tells its own story, a part of the whole.

Since retiring in 2019, Roger had to face his own mortality, living with a creeping illness that has changed how he can practice art, and which would eventually take his life. Although we did not speak much about death, Roger did share a poignant moment he had with Marshall, after art therapy had ended, when Marshall and Kerry visited him at his home:

> Two years ago, when I could still walk, but not very well. I was very doddery. There were three steps up to the studio ... when we came out I stumbled a bit. And this autistic boy, who'd been like a wild animal. A lot of people, a lot of staff found him incredibly difficult. This, child [now grown], held out his hands and stopped me from falling. ... And I could feel him holding my weight. And I thought it was a most, beautiful [Roger's voice breaks to a whisper] thing.
>
> My work, I've always thought of it as carrying children, not physically but psychologically carrying them, to perhaps, some form of safety. And he was one of the children, who I'd carried in that way and he was literally ... carrying me in a way. Holding me to save me from falling. And I think that was a very lovely thing.

When we met, Roger could no longer walk. He used a wheelchair. He struggled at times with his breathing as we talked. He said he may become tired, yet the stories flowed, and his passion was alive. We took a break midway through our meeting. Roger offered me tea and I asked if I could make it for us. His wife, Sarah, had set up cups next to the kettle. Roger directed me around the kitchen: teabags, teaspoons, milk and waste bin. When I left, he insisted I take an M&S sandwich and a chocolate bar, again sourced by Sarah before I arrived. We laughed, saying I'd get "greasy paws" all over my steering wheel. Back at the car, before I set off on my journey home, I thought about how Roger had nourished me in those few hours spent together.

Kerry said: "*If you mention Roger, Marshall smiles, it's a beautiful smile*". And Marshall added: "*Roger is like a word, a good omen for me*". However, it's not simply a fond remembrance of time spent with Roger that's held within this family. Kerry said: "*If Marshall's stressed ... we sit down and say: what would Roger say? What would Roger do?"* This short, simple phrase stopped me in my tracks. *"What would Roger do?"* I got a sense of how Marshall and Kerry had internalised a version of Roger to help them, take a pause, share understanding and move forward together, long after the work in art therapy had ended.

After we met, while I was writing up this chapter, Marshall celebrated his 21st Birthday. Roger had posted him a birthday card. To celebrate his birthday, Marshall and Kerry went to Tate Modern in London, for the day. Marshall was able to share his authority on both art and architecture with his Mum: *"I explained what it was"* referring to a particular Diego Rivera painting. Kerry said: "it was the best day I've had, ever" and "I can't wait to tell Roger".

Roger had described how humans have used art to mark their presence in the world and transcend the passage of time. *"It's almost primitive simplicity, because it's so basic. Making marks. Babies do it; they make marks. Everyone leaves marks. Bodily fluid. But also other marks that we consciously make"*. Roger has left a mark on us all. As his illness marched onwards, we didn't know he would die before the chapter was fully finished. Now, we will take him with us in our hearts.

### Conclusion

This chapter is a polaroid photograph capturing the snapshot moments of the meetings we shared. It was a deeply moving experience for me. In weaving the stories together through writing, I was struck time and again by the generosity shown to me, a stranger invited in to hear about this intimate therapeutic work. In Ireland, a seanachaí is the keeper of oral history. They are responsible for keeping the memory alive. It has been a privilege to bear a similar responsibility, in sharing the stories of Roger, Marshall and Kerry.

Moving beyond the oral tradition, we know that stories can often represent the experiences of many people. And so, these unique life stories, gathered together, contribute to an exploration of art therapy as a meaningful therapeutic tool for people with autism. More than that, they help us to see art therapy as a relational encounter which has meaning far beyond the art studio, or even the end of therapy. Although we did not plan to meet separately, in analysing the data I was struck by similar themes that emerged from very different perspectives: the importance of being artists, mutual respect, trust in the relationship and clear boundaries. I had not discussed what had happened in the different meetings.

Before finishing, it is important to also acknowledge the limitations inherent in this method. The one-off meetings provided rich data and powerful connections but could not offer the depth of a longitudinal ethnographic study for example. Additionally, while Roger, Marshall and

Kerry engaged collaboratively in reviewing the daft chapter, it is also important to note that this chapter may not fully represent their views or experiences.

Leaving this chapter now, uncertain if I will meet Marshall or Kerry again, and knowing that I cannot meet Roger again, I am left holding the power of the work we do in art therapy. Rarely as professionals do we ask about the impact or revisit clients years later to see if they remember us; maybe it's ego, maybe we shouldn't dare to hope. Yet there's a need to build genuine and affecting relationships in the present. Working in a real way with real people (hoping) to make a real difference that lasts long after therapy has ended.

## Acknowledgements

Grateful thanks to Roger, Marshall and Kerry for inviting me into their lives, for sharing their story of art therapy, then and now, and for trusting me to write this chapter. Also, sincere thanks to Sarah, Roger's wife, for her help in organising my meetings with Roger and in finalising the chapter after Roger's death.

## References

Arguile, R. (2012) 'Marking Time', *rachelalicearguile-blog*, 17 November 2012. Available at: https://rachelalicearguile-blog.tumblr.com/post/27416335467/an-area-of-work-with-which-i-have-recently-been (Accessed 1 October 2022).

Arguile, R. (1992) 'Chapter 8: Art therapy with children and adolescents', in D. Waller and A. Gilroy (eds.) *Art therapy: A handbook*. Buckingham, Philadelphia: Open University Press, pp. 140–154.

Arguile, R. (1990) 'Chapter 10: 'I show you': Children in art therapy', in T. Case and A. Dalley (eds.) *Working with children*. Hove, East Sussex: Routledge, pp. 199–216.

Case, T. and Dalley, A. (1992) *The handbook of art therapy*. Hove, East Sussex: Routledge.

Dench, S., Iphofen, R. and Huws, U. (2004) *An EU code of ethics for socio-economic research: The RESPECT project*. Available at: https://the-sra.org.uk/common/Uploaded%20files/respect%20code%20of%20ethics.pdf (Accessed on: 01/10/2022)

Douglass, B. and Moustakas, C. (1985) *Heuristic inquiry: The internal search to know*. Detroit, Michigan: Centre for Humanistic Studies.

Furman, R. (2020) 'The tenderness and vulnerability of older expatriate men: a poetic inquiry of research and autoethnographic poems', *Journal of Poetry Therapy*, 33(1), pp. 44–49. 10.1080/08893675.2020.1694222.

Gubrium, J. and Holstein, J. (2008) 'Narrative ethnography', in S. Hesse-Biber and P. Leavy (eds.) *Handbook of emergent methods*. Guilford, New York, pp. 241–264.

Hydén, L.C. and Antelius, E. (2011) 'Communicative disability and stories: Towards an embodied conception of narratives', *Health*, 15(6), pp. 588–603. 10.1177/1363459310364158.

Martin, N. (2009) 'Art therapy and autism: Overview and recommendations', *Art Therapy*, 26(4), pp. 187–190. 10.1080/07421656.2009.10129616.

Moore, S. (2020) 'A heuristic narrative inquiry on the conceptualization and cultivation of relational trust between secondary teachers and administrators'. PhD Thesis, Kansas State University, Missouri. 10.13140/RG.2.2.26211.27681.

Moustakas, C. (1990) *Heuristic research: Design methodology, and applications*. London & California: SAGE Publications, Inc.

Nyman, A., Josephsson, S. and Isaksson, G. (2012) 'Being part of an enacted togetherness: Narratives of elderly people with depression', *Journal of Aging Studies*, 26(4), pp. 410–418. 10.1016/j.jaging.2012.05.003.

Polanyi, M. (1967) *The tacit knowledge dimension*. London: Routledge & Kegan Paul.

Power, N. and Millard, E., The Lawnmowers Independent Theater Company, & Carr, C. (2022) 'Un-Labelling the Language: Exploring Labels, Jargon and Power through Participatory Arts Research with Arts Therapists and People with Learning Disabilities', *Voices: A World Forum for Music Therapy*, 22(3). 10.15 845/voices.v22i3.3391.

Rogers, C.R. (1957) 'The necessary and sufficient of therapeutic personality change', *Journal of Consulting Psychology*, 21, pp. 95–103.

Scherly, E. (2015) 'Roger Arguile: The art of looking', *ART*, 19 November 2015. Available at: https://www.meer.com/en/18336-roger-arguile (Accessed 1 October 2022).

Schweizer, C., Knorth, E. and Spreen, M. (2014) 'Art therapy with children with autism spectrum disorders: A review of clinical case descriptions on 'what works'', *The Arts in Psychotherapy*, 41(5), pp. 577–593. 10.1016/j.aip.2014.10.009.

Waller, D. and Gilroy, A (1992). *Art Therapy: A Handbook*.Open University Press.

Winnicott, D.W. (1971) *Playing & Reality*. London: Tavistock Publications.

World Health Organization (2016). *The ICD-10 classification of mental and behavioural disorders*. Genève, Switzerland: World Health Organization.

# Conclusion

## Inside-Out and Beyond

*Vicky Karkou and Supritha Aithal*

In this book, we intended to bring together important researchers and practitioners in the arts therapies who could offer the latest knowledge and understanding of how arts therapies can support the needs of clients considered as falling within the autism spectrum. However, the book offered opportunities to explore much more. For example, we covered the way arts therapies can be useful for clients whose needs are neglected, such as autistic girls (Dyer), or for those in secure care units who have been involved in criminal justice (Hackett). We have also explored needs that may receive less attention, such as sensory integration difficulties (Durrani), nonverbal autistic children (Lewis), and we have highlighted the value of focusing on kinaesthetic experiences (see Koch and Kercher). These may be areas in which arts therapies have more to offer, suggesting new ways of working and proposing exciting areas for future research.

In all these studies, the rights of children and adults on the autism spectrum are brought to the foreground, advocating for arts therapies interventions that are meaningful to autistic persons and their families. These values, and the need to bring to the foreground the voices of people with autism and their families, are articulated explicitly by Grace Thompson. They are further celebrated in Nicki Power's work in the UK where the perspectives of the client, the parent and the art therapist are highlighted. In this final chapter, we see Marshall, an autistic client who first attended art therapy as a child, forming a meaningful, important and long-lasting relationship with Roger, a pioneer art therapist in learning disabilities. The development of meaningful relationships is also discussed in other chapters in this book (e.g., Blauth); relationships via the art form are regarded as important agents of support and therapeutic value.

Philosophical stances and theoretical frameworks informing arts therapy practices have varied across the chapters. Durrani's chapter, informed by psychodynamic principles and therapist-led values, provides best practice exemplars. In other parts of the book, presumptions around professional expertise appear to give way to responsive practices that place the clients and their families at the centre of arts therapists' work and research. Many chapters in this book describe experiences of person-centred therapy (Gleason et al; Ramsden et al;) adapted to the needs and interests autistic of persons. The use of Pokemon in

DOI: 10.4324/9781003201656-19

Dyer's case study offers a good illustration of how therapy is shaped to meet the client's frame of mind. Alongside other chapters in this edited book, it encourages the therapist to come to the client rather than expect the client to conform to pre-existing notions of 'neuronormality'.

Another important issue raised in this book is the need to manualise practice within the context of health-informed research. Possibly a topic that needs further exploration in the arts therapies community, manualisation of practices is an essential requirement within studies of effectiveness that can be seen as the opposite of following the needs of the clients. Some argue that manualisation restricts practices and acts as a hindrance to the development of a therapeutic relationship. However, the chapter by Hackett offers a clear indication of how large, multi-centred, randomised, controlled trials can be accommodated with clear models of work that are repeatable without losing the flexibility required to meet clients' specific needs. Our own research (Aithal et al., 2021a) offers similar suggestions of a principle-based model rather than activity-based manuals that are developed from good practice and research and can support the needs of clients in a person-centred manner. Further discussion on this topic is certainly needed in the field of arts therapies. We expect chapters in this book will offer some useful starting points for an important debate.

Another important area the book covers is an in-depth exploration of specific techniques that are seen as relevant to meet the needs of people with autism. Mirroring, for example, is a technique extensively used by dance movement psychotherapists with a range of clients, but it may be especially important when working with people on the autistic spectrum. Intuitive value is attached to this technique. Koch and Kercher, however, provide an overall frame of important uses that is underpinned by research. Attention to this one technique within one discipline begs the question of how valuable the technique may be in other arts therapies. Combining practices and techniques across arts therapies such as music therapy and dance movement therapy (Mateos-Moreno and Atencia-Dona) or music therapy with movement (Ragone et al), and across other health interventions such as dramatherapy with speech and language therapy and play therapy (Lewis), is explored in several chapters in this book, especially in the third part of the book.

The time when solo practices were important to define disciplines and secure qualifications, professional requirements and employment appears to be giving way to collaboration and combining practices in order to meet needs and improve clinical practice. Exploring integrative practices can be a useful way forward; this will involve identifying important therapeutic factors and mechanisms of change in each of the different forms of arts therapies, as proposed in the seminal publication by an international team of arts therapists (De Witte et al., 2021). A client-specific identification of therapeutic factors may be a useful way of progressing the field, similar maybe to the systematic review by Parsons et al. (2019) followed by development work (Karkou et al., 2022; Thurston et al., 2022; Haslam et al., 2019) that led to an evidence-based multimodal creative group psychotherapy approach for depression (Omylinska-Thurston et al., 2020). This would take the work of Aithal and team that included a systematic review (2021b) and the development of an intervention model (under review) in dance movement psychotherapy for autistic children to another level, integrating best practice across arts therapies. It is possible that arts therapists from different arts therapy modalities collaborating in one session can more easily offer an integrative practice than simply splitting the session between a music and a dance movement therapist for example, as proposed in the chapter by Mateos-Moreno and Atencia-Dona.

Also referred to in this book is the role of technology as an aid to bringing knowledge, experiences and useful practices together. In the chapter by Ragone et al, music therapy was combined with movement within a technological development that aimed to expand on expressivity. In the chapter by Moo and Ho, the innovations and the limitations of using technology and tele-dance movement therapy are captured and shared, opening up a discussion about the ways technology can enable and modernise the practice of arts therapies to meet clients who may prefer, or can be further supported via, digital communication.

As highlighted in the introduction of the book, the study designs and associated perspectives are diverse. Qualitative studies vary from traditional case studies (Dyer), interviews with therapists (Moo and Ho) and parents (Bololia; Durrani; Thompson), educators (Gleeson et al) or clients, parents and therapists (Power). Some are conceptualised as narrative approach (Power), phenomenology (Mateos-Moreno and Atencia-Dona), grounded theory (Durrani, Thompson) or end of therapy evaluation (Gleeson et al). Fewer quantitative studies are reported, which perhaps highlights the need to further attend to this type of methodology. Some examples include (i) the single case study design in art therapy by Hackett, and (ii) the development of an assessment tool in music therapy by Blauth; both are making references to larger outcome studies that are either in preparation (Hackett) or already completed (Blauth). A secondary reflexive methodology that draws on theory and a small feasibility randomised controlled trial in dance movement therapy is also included (Koch and Kercher) next to a range of mixed methods approaches (Ramsden et al.; Bololia; Mateos-Moreno and Atencia-Dona).

In several chapters, the art medium is referenced not only within the clinical practice but also as a research method. The study by Power in art therapy includes the arts in descriptions of the intervention as well as using the arts as a data collection tool. In this case, visual artwork and poems are used respectively. The use of emotion stones as a routine initial assessment tool and as a research method/evaluation technique is described in the study by Ramsden et al. It is therefore clear that the arts are valued as a means to engage, transform and communicate change. They carry information that can be treated as data allowing participants in the study who are non-verbal to find ways in which they can share their wishes, needs and experiences of the arts therapies process and outcomes. More studies capturing client experiences are needed that do not rely simply on carers' views. Arts-based methods, the bread and butter of arts therapies practice, offer the promising potential to enable clients' voices to become loud and clear. Collaborative research with clients (in the UK this is often referred to as Patient and Public Involvement and Engagement practice) is also needed, a practice that is increasingly becoming an essential requirement in funded research. Collaborative research can allow for the adoption of diverse types of research methodologies without risking the generation of findings that do not serve the autism community, i.e., those intending to benefit in the first place.

Overall, the studies presented in this book highlight several important outcomes, as well as individual and group processes for participants on the autism spectrum in arts therapies. These interventions not only reduce difficulties such as general anxiety and psychological distress, as discussed by Hackett, but can also build personal strengths and resilience (Blauth). Perceived and measured outcomes from the perspectives of clients, therapists, caregivers and educators are grouped under the following domains:

**Social and Communication:** behaviours and skills that enable the building and strengthening of the quality of relationships through enjoyable interactions (Dyer; Thompson; Blauth; Lewis; Gleason et al; Moo and Ho) provide motivation to engage in therapy, and outside of therapy (Bololia; Moo and Ho) give a sense of identity and autonomy (Bololia), increase verbal and non verbal vocabulary (Lewis; Mateos-Moreno and Atencia-Doña) and establish boundaries (Power; Durrani).

**Psychological** (Emotional and Cognitive): assist in the development of insight and emotional literacy, expressing emotions and needs (Ramsden et al.), strengthening protective factors including resilience (Blauth), reducing anxiety, loneliness and psychological distress (Hackett; Mateos-Moreno and Atencia-Doña), maintaining wellbeing, positive feelings (Moo and Ho), internal self-reflection and new perspectives.

**Physical and Sensory:** providing physical proximity/closeness in space (promoting, sensory regulation, integration and self-soothing techniques (Durrani; Bololia).

Empathy is discussed by Koch and Kercher, who argue that further consideration is needed to establish whether the structural features of autism, such as empathy, can indeed be positively affected by arts therapies and, if yes, how. This, along with the outcomes listed above, appears to be an important topic for future outcome studies to provide conclusive evidence of the benefits of arts therapies for this client population. Studies with follow-up measures are also needed to show the degree to which these benefits are sustainable. Also, as implied in different parts of this book, further work is needed to find out whether clinical observations are transferable to everyday life, linking people on the autism spectrum with their families and their wider social circles. It is possible that specific creative and non verbal techniques can be shared amongst families and friends who are willing to meet people with autism where they are and interact in their preferred ways of interacting, i.e., visually, bodily and digitally. It may also be possible to offer therapeutic support to carers vulnerable to burnout, as argued in some of our studies with caregivers (Aithal et al., 2019, 2020, 2021c).

In all cases, based on the studies included in this book alone, positive contributions are noticeable, suggesting that the arts therapies can indeed support people on the autism spectrum and their families, enable wider social movements and connections. We are convinced that the gentle, person-centred, creative approaches often inherent in arts therapies practice can offer opportunities for respecting and accepting the differences and support that will lead to the growth of a range of abilities and strengths, beautifully captured in the following quote and depicted in Figure 15.1:

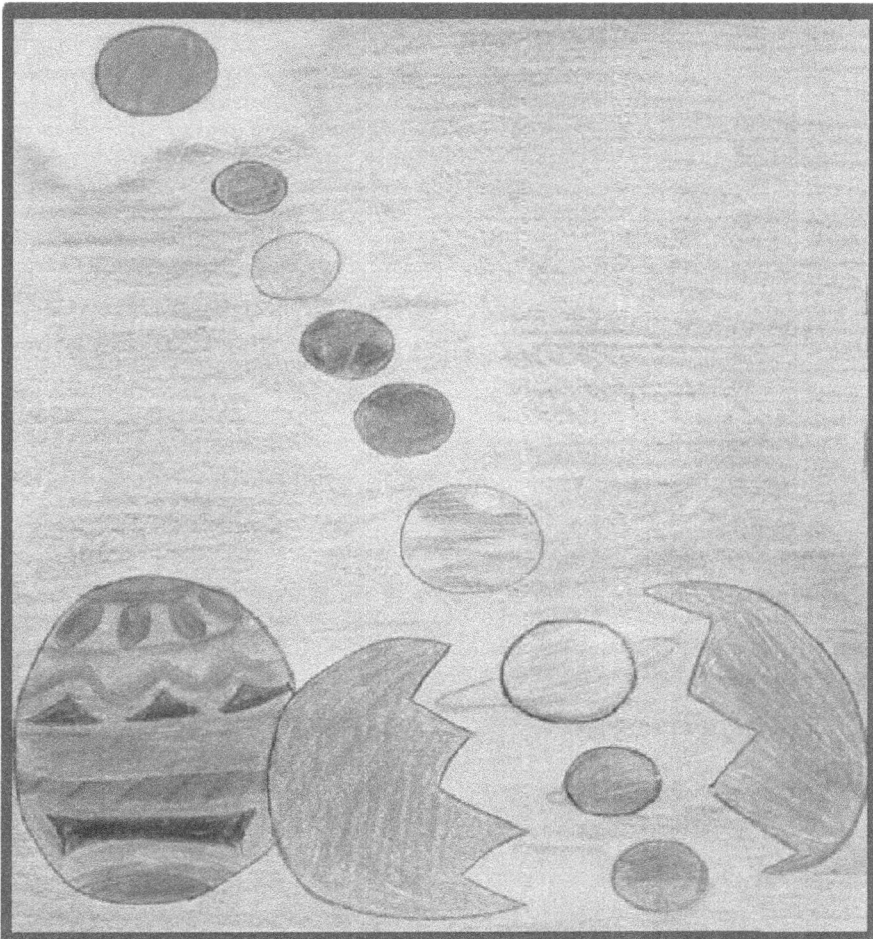

*Figure 15.1* Inside-out and beyond by Anvitha S. Rao (13 years) from Sarayu Kala Kuteera, Bengaluru

If an egg is broken by an outside force, *life ends*. If broken by an inside force, *life begins*.

– (Anonymous)

We believe arts therapies can nurture the potential of an individual to manifest from inside-out and beyond. Through this book, *Colourful Hatchlings* glimpses of how growth can be facilitated through arts therapies are offered, making an important and research-informed contribution regarding the approaches and benefits of arts therapies for people on the autism spectrum.

## References

Aithal, S., Karkou, V., Mariswamy, P. and Kuppusamy, G. (2019) 'Backing the backbones – A feasibility study on the effectiveness of dance movement psychotherapy on parenting stress in caregivers of children with Autism Spectrum Disorders', *The Arts in Psychotherapy*, 64, pp. 69–76. 10.1016/j.aip.2019.04.003.

Aithal, S., Karkou, V., Mariswamy, P. and Kuppusamy, G. (2020) 'Resilience enhancement in parents of children with an autism spectrum disorder through dance movement psychotherapy', *The Arts in Psychotherapy*, 71, 101708. 10.1016/j.aip.2020.101708.

Aithal, S., Karkou, V.V., Makris, S., Karaminis, T. and Powell, J. (2021a) 'A dance movement psychotherapy intervention for the wellbeing of children with autism spectrum disorders: a pilot intervention study', *Frontiers in Psychology*, 12, p. 2672. 10.3389/fpsyg.2021.588418.

Aithal, S., Moula, Z., Karkou, V., Karaminis, T., Powell, J. and Makris, S. (2021b) 'A systematic review of the contribution of dance movement psychotherapy towards the well-being of children with autism spectrum disorders', *Frontiers in Psychology*, 4238. 10.3389/fpsyg.2021.719673.

Aithal, S., Karkou, V., Makris, S., Karaminis, T. and Powell, J. (2021c) 'Impact of dance movement psychotherapy on the wellbeing of caregivers of children with autism spectrum disorder', *Public Health*, 10.1016/j.puhe.2021.09.018.

De Witte, M., Orkibi, H., Zarate, R., Karkou, V., Sajnani, S., Malhotra, B., Ho, R.T.H., Kaimal, G., Baker, F.A. and Koch, S.C. (2021) 'From therapeutic factors to mechanisms of change in the creative arts therapies: A scoping review', *Frontiers in Psychology*. 10.3389/fpsyg.2021.678397.

Haslam, S., Parsons, A.S., Omylinska-Thurston, J., Nair, K., Harlow, J., Lewis, J., Dubrow- Marshall, L., Thurston, S., Griffin, J. and Karkou, V. (2019) 'Arts for the Blues – A new creative psychological therapy for depression – A pilot workshop report', *Perspectives in Public Health*, 139(3), pp. 137–146. 10.1177/1757913919826599.

Karkou, V., Omylinska-Thurston, J., Parsons, A., Nair, K., Starkey, J., Haslam, S., Thurston, S. and Dubrow-Marshall, L. (2022) 'Bringing Creative Psychotherapies to Primary NHS Mental Health Services in the UK: A Feasibility Study on Patient and Staff Experiences of Arts for the Blues Workshops Delivered at Improving

Access to Psychological Therapies (IAPT) services', *Counselling and Psychotherapy Research*, https://onlinelibrary.wiley.com/doi/10.1002/capr.12544.

Omylinska-Thurston, J., Karkou, V., Parson, A., Dudley-Swarbrick, I., Haslam, S., Lewis, J., Nair, K., Dubrow-Marshall, L. and Thurston, S. (2020) 'Arts for the Blues: The development of a new evidence-based creative group psychotherapy for depression', *Counselling and Psychotherapy Research*. 10.1002/capr.12373.

Parsons, A., Omylinska-Thurston, J., Karkou, V., Harlow, J., Haslam, S., Hobson, J. Nair, K., Dubrow-Marshall, L., Thurston, S. and Griffin, J. (2019) 'Arts for the blues – A new creative psychological therapy for depression', *British Journal of Guidance and Counselling*, 48(1), pp. 5–20. 10.1080/03069885.2019.1633459.

Thurston, S., Griffin, J., Davismoon, S., Omylinska-Thurston, J. and Karkou, V. (2022) 'Dancing the Blues: An interdisciplinary collaboration between artists and therapists', *Journal of Applied Arts and Health*, 10.1386/jaah_00107_1.

# Index